MAINTAINING RECOVERY FROM EATING DISORDERS

MAINTAINING RECOVERY FROM EATING DISORDERS

Avoiding Relapse and Recovering Life

NAOMI FEIGENBAUM

Foreword by Rebekah Bardwell Doweyko

Jessica Kingsley *Publishers*
London and Philadelphia

First published in 2012
by Jessica Kingsley Publishers
116 Pentonville Road
London N1 9JB, UK
and
400 Market Street, Suite 400
Philadelphia, PA 19106, USA

www.jkp.com

Library of Congress Cataloging in Publication Data
Feigenbaum, Naomi.
  Maintaining recovery from eating disorders : avoiding relapse and recovering
life / Naomi Feigenbaum ; foreword by Rebekah Bardwell Doweyko.
    p. cm.
  Includes index.
  ISBN 978-1-84905-815-5 (alk. paper)
  1. Feigenbaum, Naomi--Health. 2. Eating disorders--Relapse--Prevention. 3.
Eating disorders--Patients--Rehabilitaiton. I. Title.
  RC552.E18F45 2012
  616.85'2605--dc22
                                    2011010172

British Library Cataloguing in Publication Data
A CIP catalogue record for this book is available from the British Library

ISBN 9781849058155

Printed and bound in Great Britain

Dedicated to my Mom and Dad
with love and admiration

You are the best parents in the world and I love
you with all my heart. You inspire me to follow my
dreams and define my own success. Over the years
you have created and sustained a warm, fun, and
loving family, and you continue to be there for each
of us. People say it's a hard day when you realize that
your parents aren't superheroes. I wouldn't know
because I'm twenty-three years old and my parents
still are superheroes. I suspect you always will be.

CONTENTS

Author's Note

While this book indicates signs and symptoms of eating disorders and demonstrates healthy coping skills for recovery, it is not meant to take the place of professional guidance or therapy. Recovery from an eating disorder is not something you should attempt on your own. It is my hope that this book will aid in readers' recoveries, and help their loved ones better understand the process and how they can be supportive. Use this book as a springboard for self-discovery and hope. Take what you need and leave the rest. There is no "right way."

Each man and woman who so bravely shares their story in this book has achieved recovery in their own way. There are a limited number of ways to have an eating disorder, but there are an infinite number of ways to be in recovery.

I thank all those who have given permission to use their stories, their names have been changed to protect their confidentiality.

FOREWORD

When Naomi asked me to write the foreword for her latest book, saying I felt honored would be an understatement. It is an honor and a privilege to write this foreword for many reasons. When I began working in the eating disorder field just over ten years ago, it was very difficult to recommend books for bibliotherapy, a useful treatment intervention for various addictions and mental illnesses. According to the Encyclopedia of Mental Disorders, "Bibliotherapy is an adjunct to psychological treatment that incorporates appropriate books or other written materials, usually intended to be read outside of psychotherapy sessions, into the treatment regimen." You see, the problem was that most books written by those who suffered from eating disorders unfortunately spent a great deal of the book focusing on (in great detail) the symptoms of the eating disorder. Although this may have been a powerful coping tool for the writer, for the reader, this often gave them new ideas, tricks, and ways to avoid getting caught by parents, spouses, and clinicians. Furthermore, books focusing on eating disorder symptoms, although well meaning, often did little to empower one toward recovery, and instead, often made the situation worse, as the reader readily identified with the symptoms and the desperation of the writer. This was unfortunately not the area of expertise the reader needed to focus on, as he or she clearly already had a grasp of the symptoms of an eating disorder and needed to learn how to do recovery.

Fortunately, in 2004, Jenni Schaefer published the bestselling book *Life Without Ed*. Finally, a book focusing on recovery was here! I believe that Naomi has followed in Jenni's footsteps with her first book *One Life*, offering a candid look at eating disorder treatment. Naomi writes honestly about her intense experiences in her preliminary treatment and recovery in residential treatment at the Renfrew Center in Coconut Creek, Florida.

Most of the books written in the past about eating disorders seem to focus primarily on anorexia nervosa, secondarily on bulimia nervosa, and very rarely on binge eating disorder (BED) or ED NOS (eating disorder not otherwise specified). Ironically, BED and ED NOS (this diagnosis is given when the symptoms do not fit neatly into the anorexia or bulimia box) are the most commonly occurring types of eating disorders, yet are the least likely to be covered by insurance companies, and are the least identified in literature, thus perpetuating the shame, guilt, and secrecy associated with these debilitating disorders. In *Maintaining Recovery from Eating Disorders* the reader will be introduced to several struggles and successes depicted in the personal stories of men and women struggling with a variety of eating disorder symptoms.

If you are reading this, it is most likely because you have been fortunate enough to have purchased or been given *Maintaining Recovery from Eating Disorders*, the second novel by the dynamic and empowering Naomi Feigenbaum who chronicles her continued experience in recovery as well as the recovery experiences from men and women of a variety of ages, cultures, races, and ranges of specific eating disorder struggles.

Maintaining Recovery from Eating Disorders works to help those at varying levels in their recovery, answering that often perplexing question, "okay so here I am in recovery, now what?" Naomi also focuses on that difficult transition from treatment to the "real world" that if not done successfully, often leads to relapse.

Additionally, the reader will discover helpful ways to explore the "new world" that is sometimes unrecognizable after being entrenched in an eating disorder for many years. *Maintaining Recovery from Eating Disorders* helps empower the reader to continue their journey of self-discovery and emotional growth. Emotional growth may, in fact, be one of the key elements in recovery. Over the past eleven years, I have often observed that those who struggle with eating disorders (and other addictions) clearly display what seems like a stunted emotional maturity. On several occasions, distraught patients have sat in my office, sobbing or venting, saying, "I don't know what is wrong with me! I feel like I am seven years old right now!" My usual response is, "well maybe, emotionally, that *is*, exactly how old you are." Initially, this doesn't usually go over so well. However, after a thorough explanation, the sentiment is often right on the money. You see, at the point one begins to act on addictive behaviors meant to numb intense "negative" feelings, the ability to process and learn how to cope with these feelings is halted. As a result, these feelings remain buried, misunderstood, confusing, and begin to build underneath the skin as if they have been literally "swept under the carpet." If someone has been using food or exercise as a means to avoid feelings that are uncomfortable or feelings that have been deemed unacceptable, it is likely that she will stunt her emotional growth – being unable to communicate or to cope with life. Thus, she turns to the eating disorder to communicate and cope for her, which only deepens the vicious cycle leading her down a path of self-destruction.

Maintaining Recovery from Eating Disorders also focuses on several other essentials in recovering one's emotional maturity, including relationships, spirituality, and trauma. Naomi highlights the importance of individuation: developing integrity and one's own core beliefs, values, opinions and expressing them. Other central topics are discussed such as complacency, grief and loss, the importance of an appropriate treatment team, boundaries, triggers, and, of course, body image.

Two of the most common themes I hear in treating those with eating disorders are triggers and body image. If I had a dime for every time a patient shouted, "trigger!" throughout treatment, I would be a very rich woman. Often times, I see parents and clinicians trying to allay the trigger and provide a "trigger-free" environment. In an attempt to ease the patient's struggle, I feel we miss a very important opportunity for emotional growth. You see, the world is *full* of triggers and the patient needs to learn how to effectively cope with the ones that are unavoidable. *Maintaining Recovery from Eating Disorders* aids the reader in how to cope effectively with daily triggers, again furthering emotional development.

The other common theme I have heard woven into the exclamations of those in treatment is regarding body image and the idea that "it is the first to come, and it will be the last to go." Although this may be reassuring at the time, it is entirely false. Any human being on this planet on any given day may experience negativity about his or her body. Now, is there a difference between pathological negative body image and "normal" negative body image? Yes. But expecting to love every inch of your body every minute of every day is unrealistic. We all have bad body image days. It is the power you give to your bad body image day that counts.

In addition, Naomi discusses nutrition and defines essential concepts such as emotional eating, mechanical eating, and mindful eating. Most of those who struggle with eating disorders have lost the ability to discern hunger or fullness, to identify correct portion size, or even to allow the taste of the food to be acknowledged and enjoyed. Eating disorders may not be "about the food," but too often the nutritional element of a sustained recovery is ignored. Thanks to Naomi, this is no longer the case.

The road to learning how to eat when you are hungry and to stop when you are full has been paved.

Working with Naomi has been akin to what I often hear other proud therapists refer to as "the reason why we do this work." When I began graduate school over ten years ago, I reflected on what my expectations were of myself in this field that some describe as difficult and trying. Upon reflection, what I came up with was that if I could reach (notice I said reach, not cure) just one person, and guide them toward making positive changes in their life, it would all be worth it. Well, Naomi, if someone had told me that I would have achieved my goal so early in my career, I would have accused them of lying. You are such a special young woman, and my wish for you, and for whomever is reading this foreword, is that you continue (or start) to see in yourself what others see. That you continue to explore your feelings no matter how difficult, and that you begin (or continue) to be willing to form your own opinions and make your own mistakes. That you use your "powers" for good and not evil. And, finally, that you continue this rollercoaster of a journey called life with patience and tolerance, living life on life's terms. I know you can do it. All of you have the power and strength somewhere inside yourselves to recover – for good! If I had to name one thing that I believe has aided Naomi in her journey to and in recovery, it would be her ability to accept and apply feedback. I believe that as you read this book, you will also be able to connect with Naomi's incredible ability to empower those struggling to achieve what she has, and continues to work hard to maintain: the belief that it is possible. That it is simple, just not easy. Naomi, I am so proud of all you have accomplished. I respect and admire you greatly. You are just as amazing in your struggles as you are in your successes, since in the final analysis, it is our struggles that lead us to success – and without which we would have neither insight nor confidence.

Rebekah Bardwell Doweyko, LMHC

ACKNOWLEDGEMENTS

First and foremost I thank my parents, Meshullam (Mesh) and Elene (Motheroo) Feigenbaum for everything you do. I cannot think of two people more dedicated and devoted to family than you.

I also want to thank my sisters and brother. Adina, Sarah (Lolly), and Joseph (Yoey), you are all awesome. I can't think of people so different and yet so similar than the four of us. I know that wherever we are we will always be close. I especially want to thank Lolly (with heart) because without you there would be no Chapters 1 and 2. I exaggerate, but not by much. Thank you for your countless hours spent transcribing my interview tapes for this project. And of course, I can't forget to thank Skittles, Taffy, and Mandi. (Okay, and the frogs!)

To everyone who helped me – and continues to help me – on my journey of recovery: Thank you with all my heart. I am especially grateful to Rabbi Burnstein for your dedication and commitment to helping me get well and stay well, never giving up and always being there for me and for my family, and in truth for everyone in your congregation and greater community. You are a gem and a key player in the lives of many.

Thank you to Rebekah Bardwell Doweyko for being a world class therapist (I completely mean that). You've helped me grow in ways I never imagined before I met you. Thank you for writing such a beautiful Foreword. Thank you to all the professionals who devoted time and guidance to this project. Thank you to the Renfrew Center, The Center for Intuitive Eating, and the Cleveland Center for Eating Disorders for the great work you do to help people better their lives. A heartfelt thank you to the individuals whose stories run throughout this book. Your sharing will help countless others and for that you deserve all the thanks in the world.

I am sincerely grateful for my fantastic team at Jessica Kingsley Publishers. It is a joy and a pleasure to work with all of you – from editing to production to marketing and everything in between. Lily Morgan, thank you for showing me the ropes in the publishing world, for believing in my work, and for presenting me with the tremendous opportunity to spread my message of empowerment on a grand scale. Lisa Clark, I enjoyed working with you on *One Life* and it's been wonderful to work with you on another project. Thank you both for your guidance and for always being available to answer my questions. Thank you to Jessica Kingsley for "trusting the process" and setting my creativity free! Thank you for providing me with such an opportunity and for incorporating my input into the final product. JKP is an author's dream.

I also want to take a moment to thank my graduate school advisor – and mentor – at Florida Atlantic University, Dr. Paul Peluso. You have been a guiding force for me from the day I set foot on the FAU campus. Thank you for helping me develop my skills, clarify my passion, and ultimately set myself free. It's an ongoing process and I'm not quite there... yet. You are an incredible source of inspiration and wisdom and I am honored to be your student.

Introduction

The Journey Beyond Eating Disorders

After achieving some level of recovery from an eating disorder, many people find themselves asking, "Now what?" There are many books and resources geared toward individuals trying to ease up on symptom use – such as binging, purging, restricting, or a number of other unhealthy behaviors associated with eating disorders – but shockingly few for those who are actively in recovery. Perhaps even fewer resources exist for those seeking not only to maintain long-term physical, mental, and emotional health, but also to continue their journeys of discovery and growth.

Eating disorders never develop in a vacuum and often serve as a form of pseudo-protection. When you focus on your physical eating disorder, either by using your symptoms or trying not to use your symptoms, you are naturally *not* focusing on the underlying issues. That isn't to say that stopping your symptom use isn't a valuable use of your time and effort. Of *course* it is important, but it is only the beginning of true recovery.

Most recovery work occurs *in recovery itself.* Only once you cease to rely on eating disorder symptoms can you truly face up to your underlying issues. *Maintaining Recovery from Eating Disorders* addresses a number of different areas in which you may struggle – such as relationships, spirituality, and trauma. As you read this book, try to focus on your own situation. You are not in competition with anyone. You may not struggle with everything mentioned in this book. You may also have struggles that are not addressed. It is important to remember that you are a unique individual with your own inner world and outer life experiences, and just as weight and body shape do not define your worth, neither do your struggles.

The book offers a fresh outlook on several common challenges faced by those in recovery from eating disorders and presents the practical guidance and suggestions of several treatment professionals. This book will also introduce you to a number of men and women in recovery, providing a glimpse into their lives as they maintain recovery each moment:

Introducing Jessica, twenty

I am hard-working, dedicated, a leader, funny, and extremely sarcastic. I was confident in my athletic abilities up until my eating disorder began around the age of sixteen. I know I'm different than many other people my age in the sense that I don't drink, smoke, or do drugs. I've been somewhat active in church since I was sixteen (how ironic). I currently play golf at a Division II school and couldn't design a school where I would be happier than I am right now.

Jessica's story

After my family moved to Georgia I immediately became self-conscious of my looks because of the tan, thin, blonde girls that seemed to overtake my new town. I started cutting out certain foods completely from my diet. I lost a few pounds and that made me feel good about myself. My senior year of high school was when my life came crashing down. My boyfriend died in a terrible accident. He had a few drinks and went for a drive without his seatbelt. Life hasn't been the same since. I started to skip lunch at this point, mainly because I would be hiding somewhere crying during lunch. Everything would remind me of my boyfriend. People would make the tiniest comments and they would set me off. I focused more on softball and began running everyday to try to get in shape for college softball. I wanted to be fast and the more weight I lost, the faster I would get. Weight became a huge obsession for me. I started weighing myself several times a day. I realized I had a problem by this point and had lost control of my life. A week after my eighteenth birthday I went into a partial hospitalization program. Four months later I went into Renfrew. Exactly one month after I discharged myself against medical advice, I had to go back to a partial hospitalization program about three hours from where I live. Exactly two months after my initial discharge date from Renfrew brought my second "first day" at Renfrew. Sixty days later I discharged, having completed the program. I was happier than I felt in four years. Things that have helped me during this process have been the realization that I *do* have something to live for and that I'm not a failure at life because I became anorexic. I put things in a bigger perspective compared to the world. How could a certain weight be the worst thing to ever happen to me? I accepted that I wasn't a failure for going to treatment so many times for so long, that my recovery is my own individual process, and that even Superman has kryptonite.

Introducing Lexi, twenty-three

At twenty-three years old, a part of me still feels fifteen while another part feels as though I have lived a lifetime. The great thing is that I still have a lifetime to go and the energy of a fifteen-year-old; a lifetime of experiences, learning and growing, laughing and loving. As a graduate student working toward earning my doctor of physical therapy degree at Creighton University in Omaha, Nebraska, I am developing the skills needed to not only help people heal physically but also how to meet them where they are emotionally and to avoid preconceived judgments about their conditions and diseases. While school keeps me extremely busy between the academic, club and leadership positions I hold, I try to balance my time with other things I enjoy – such as playing intramural sports, running, photography, being active in my church as a youth leader and participant in a program called Celebrate Recovery, and having a little sister in the Big Brothers/Big Sisters program. I love my friends and family dearly; without them I would not be where or who I am today.

Lexi's story

My story involves one of struggles, achievements, falling but picking myself back up, trials, hurts, pain – and a lot of growth. The seeds for anorexia nervosa were planted when I was young and grew into my senior year of high school. During my first three years of college, I had times when I acted on my eating disorder and times when I didn't. During my junior year I hit rock bottom. Anorexia, over-exercising and purging, became my life. Food, lack of food or exercising was all I could think about. My spiritual self was gone. I was isolating myself from friends who were trying to support me in every way possible. Self-harm became another unhealthy coping mechanism. I began my journey of recovery at Renew, an outpatient clinic in Olathe, Kansas. I started to slowly break through the walls I had built around myself and around my heart. I built trust with my therapist, honesty with my dietitian and openness with my therapy group. I traveled home for therapy most weekends during my senior year of college. It was tedious at the time, but very necessary. Building relationships and forming new ones, finding out what real friendships were, discovering myself, rejuvenating my relationship with my parents and having a brother who constantly supported me has made all the hard times worth it. I'm not going to say that recovery is all flowers and sunshine. There are some rainy days built in, however, those rainy days always come to an end and they bring about new flowers. Recovery is worth it. Life is worth it. Life is a gift, a journey, and something I am so glad to have back.

Introducing Taylor, twenty-eight

I am creative and funny. At least I hope so because otherwise I just entertain myself. I love computers and rather enjoy music. I'm definitely outgoing and treat my friends with kindness, caring, and compassion. Sometimes I'm stubborn, but that works to my benefit. If I had to pick two words to describe me, I would pick "creative" and "passionate" because those are the two things I keep together with me in everything I do.

Taylor's story

My grandmother died when I was eight years old and my family fell apart. Two years later I ended up in a school where I had no friends, while my family experienced horrible medical drama. It wasn't long before my eating disorder developed. But the frustrating part was that I didn't fit into any "box" – there was no definitive category to explain my symptoms – and thus I struggled to get the help I needed. I was told time and time again that I wasn't really so sick. And this from supposed eating disorder experts! After long, hard years of knocking on doors that wouldn't open, I finally came to the conclusion that the only one who could truly validate me is *me*. My story is one of loss and neglect, but I am not a victim – I am a survivor. My stubborn nature leads me to never give up. But I also know when to be flexible. When I was sixteen, I wrote in my journal that, "I, Taylor B. Lancaster, will one day be an actress and know that I followed my dream." At nineteen I revised it, writing, "I either want to be a lawyer or play one on TV." And now, at twenty-eight, I believe that if I could do anything that would allow me to combine my creativity, my writing, my computer skills, and my desire to help people, then I would be set. And poor. (There's my humor again!)

Introducing Aurora, twenty-five

I am a deeply spiritual person. The times I struggle the most in life, with anything – including my eating disorder – are the times when I'm spiritually disconnected. Even though I was brought up with certain values and traditions, and even though I still cherish and uphold much of what my family has given me, I also am learning to be my own person and find my own path. It takes a lot of trial and error but I'm on my way.

Aurora's story

My story has been one of grief and loss but also one of faith and meaning. I've been through more than my fair share of hardship, tragically losing my father and my brother at young ages. I've been in abusive relationships and at times almost completely lost track of who I am. During times of ambivalence I learned to turn to those I trust most. I am blessed to have a unique and special relationship with my therapist. She was the one who broke the news to me that my father passed away while I was in treatment. She helped me cope with the darkness and begin seeking out the light. I am very grateful to have her in my life. There were definitely dark times in my past, but I know that my true self is creative, connected, bright, and spiritual. I thrive on energy – on my inner power and on the power of the universe.

Introducing Andrew, thirty-five

I am a husband and a father of two wonderful boys living in Dublin, Ireland. I work as an engineer and have my own personal training business. I love cinema and hiking and clubbing and spending time with my family. It doesn't matter what we do, I just enjoy being with them. We like nature and being outdoors. The eating disorder that once ruled my life is gone. I consider myself recovered. Not "in recovery" but actually "recovered." If you don't believe that recovery is possible then how are you going to do it? What's the motivation to fight for it? You have to believe there's an end to all of it. I can't bear the thought of going back. I could never re-live those horrendous experiences. I'm not saying life is a bed of roses now either, but rather than cope via the eating disorder, I have the skills now to cope with whatever comes my way. I don't need the eating disorder anymore.

If I could say one thing to people who are struggling it would be that there is no need to be ashamed. I always come back to the expression that no man is an island. Reach out for help. Life after recovery is fantastic. People are afraid of their own potential. What life is like in recovery becomes scary. When you're stuck in an eating disorder you have no comprehension of what life is like without that. Life has a lot to offer if you let go of the eating disorder. My life has become a series of stepping stones. As I become more courageous and realize what life has to offer, there is more that I, in turn, can contribute.

Andrew's story

When I was nineteen I realized that I was in serious trouble. I needed help. I wanted help. A plan to work out and get fit had gotten out of control and my doctor told me I had anorexia and needed to seek help from a therapist. The therapist helped me a little bit but I spent the following ten years recovering and relapsing, recovering and relapsing. It wasn't until I was twenty-nine that I finally attained full recovery. My eating disorder kept me completely detached from myself. It was a means of avoiding myself. Working out kept me from thinking the thoughts in my head – kept me from thinking about how I hated myself.

I'm a completely different person now. I have a good life. I have a wife and kids. I have confidence. I know that I'm good at the things I do and I don't need to prove myself to other people. I accept myself for who I am. It was a slow process and there were no individual aha moments. I used to have extremely high, unrealistic expectations. It was an issue I had to deal with in therapy. The center that I recovered at ultimately gave me back the power to live my life.

Introducing Korrie, nineteen

Probably my greatest strength is that I am real. I don't blab my secrets to the world or anything, but I don't hide who I am, either. Sometimes, especially when I'm not in a good mood, it's obvious to other people. A lot of times I wear my emotions on my sleeve. Some people are turned off by it, but I have my close friends who appreciate my honest and real sharing. I'm extremely loyal and stick up for my friends.

I'm also a very determined and motivated person. Even when I struggle, I struggle honestly and with a fierce determination to overcome my obstacles. I also try very hard to treat everyone with kindness. I don't intentionally play mind games. I try to always stick up for what I believe in, even when it's not popular.

Korrie's story

If I could redo the past years and my treatment, I definitely would because I didn't take advantage of everything I could have. Even though I did a lot of important work, there is still a lot more that I could have done. I never thought that I would go back into my old mindset, but lately I have had many struggles. It seems I also have swapped symptoms. It's hard because I've been in recovery for so long that it's embarrassing to admit slips. But if there's one thing I've learned it's that honesty keeps me on the path of recovery. I try very hard to take my own advice, and my biggest piece of advice is to *take advantage of every opportunity*. Comply with the professionals on your team. An eating disorder is a serious illness, and even though we think we know best, most of the time our treatment teams know better. Even though it's very hard, I'm learning to let people in. My team, my family, my friends. It's a leap of faith sometimes, but you have to trust people.

Each of these individuals has struggled and triumphed over eating disordered behaviors, turning their biggest weaknesses into their biggest strengths. They have had ups and downs and the highway of life continues to present roadblocks and other hazards, but they continue to navigate the road without the "help" of their eating disorders or any other backseat driver.

Food and weight and other numbers should only take up a small part of your life. Thinking about it more than that takes away from your real life. Sometimes it's easier to subconsciously avoid life by slipping into a numbing zone such as an eating disorder, because then you are mentally not present. This book aims to help you discover your own roadmap – your unique insights and passions and ultimately a life for which you will be mentally present because you won't want to miss it.

This is not a book about eating disorders. It is a book about real life, the journey *beyond* eating disorders...

Chapter 1

Making a Smooth Transition

"I always tried to do everything alone,
I had to give that up. Surrender."

– Aurora

After leaving treatment for an eating disorder, it is a challenge to maintain recovery. Common struggles range from applying newly-learned coping skills to everyday life situations to full-blown "culture shock," as is often the case for those leaving residential and other more intensive forms of treatment. You may also face a variety of other challenges that are uniquely yours. The important thing is to remember that struggles are opportunities for growth. You have the ability not only to remain in recovery through a struggle, but also to use each struggle to *enhance* your recovery.

It is very common for people leaving treatment to feel a sense of insecurity. You may question your readiness to leave. You may feel a lack of confidence in your ability to lead a healthy life outside of treatment. You may even feel afraid and wonder what a life in recovery *is,* especially if you have been consumed by your eating disorder for many years. You are likely to face many struggles after treatment, both big and small. That is perfectly okay and in fact, it is a part of the recovery process. Confidence develops over time. According to Rebekah Bardwell Doweyko, LMHC and director and founder of the Center for Intuitive Eating at the Hollywood Pavilion in Florida, the only way to build true confidence is to allow yourself to struggle and appropriately manage your struggles – by allowing yourself to feel emotion throughout your struggles, even difficult emotion; reaching out for support; and using healthy coping skills.

If you numb yourself through your struggles, refusing to feel, you deny yourself opportunities for emotional growth. Rebekah explains in her Foreword to this book that many men and women she sees in treatment have stunted their emotional growth so that, on an emotional level, they act and feel much younger than they truly are. It is yet another handicap produced by eating disorders.

Many individuals with eating disorders engage in unhealthy behaviors in an attempt to numb themselves and their feelings and many people describe the journey of recovery as a journey from childhood to adulthood. Rebekah explains, "Numbing behaviors most accurately reflect the warmth of infancy." In infancy all of your needs must be met by others, but for many people infancy and childhood are disrupted. This can happen in a number of ways. Sometimes in families with children close in age, an infant's needs may take priority over a slightly older child's needs. If a child comes from a large family or has a sibling with special needs, a similar situation can arise in which the child's needs are not being met fully or quickly enough. Other disrupting situations can involve children being raised by grieving parents or parents who are distracted by any number of stressors in their own lives. All of these instances result in a child's needs being set aside, at least temporarily, because at that moment somebody else's needs are deemed more important. Left to their own devices, these children sometimes resort to numbing behaviors reminiscent of an earlier stage of development.

This is a pattern that can occur at any stage of life in which your needs are not met. An eating disorder involves many familiar, childlike patterns. My memories during my sickest moments have a sort of hazy, childlike quality to them, almost the way I remember my seventh birthday or my second grade school play. When a person becomes ill through lack of nutrition their entire being is affected and others are forced to care for them. On a subconscious level this can occur for a multitude of reasons but it is almost always an attempt to meet a need that person has – it can be an attempt to reclaim a lost childhood, to get even with distant parents or other significant people in their lives, or to fill an emotional void.

Taylor

Within a one month period, Taylor's mother broke her ankle in twelve places, her brother had the first of five brain surgeries, and her father was hospitalized for a suicide attempt. Taylor was the only member of her family who was not in the hospital. In fact, the rest of her family was at the same hospital! They frequented the hospital so much during that year that one time when her parents visited the hospital café, a nurse had to ask who was visiting who. On another occasion, when Taylor's brother was wheeled in for his third brain surgery, he asked, "Can we do this in surgery room three? That seems to be a lucky one for me."

With both of Taylor's parents effectively disabled and coping with the fact that their son was quite possibly dying, Taylor was left to fend for herself emotionally. To make matters worse, she had just transferred to a new school where she had no friends to help *her* cope with the horrendous drama in her life.

It was precisely during this timeframe that Taylor began experimenting with eating disorder symptoms. Her reasons were twofold. Subconsciously it was a way for her to put her feelings all in one place. It forced her to think of something other than real life. On the other hand, Taylor's developing eating disorder was a way for her to seek attention from her family – a way for her to communicate that her needs were not being met and that she was hurting. Unfortunately her family remained unresponsive to her cries for help.

"The ante was up so high, so many times, that unless my heart ran out at exactly that moment, I still wouldn't get the attention," says Taylor. "My mom was dying and so that took precedence all the time. She 'won.'"

At a certain point, Taylor got up the strength and courage to flat out ask her mother if she could go to therapy. Her mother dismissed her, saying, "I'm dying right now!"

Taylor sadly replied, "I kind of am, too."

Soon Taylor's mother was gone. That wasn't going to change. Her rocky relationship with her father wasn't going to change, either. It took a long time for Taylor to come to terms with the fact that her needs were not met, and would not be met, by her biological family. If she was going to recover and live a healthy life, she would have to summon the strength herself, just as she had when she took that first step of sharing her need for therapy with her mother. Although her pleas for help were disregarded by her parents, Taylor would still embark on the journey to wellness. Waiting for her family to step up was like waiting for her mom to come back to life – no matter how much her heart ached for it, it would never happen.

In recovery today Taylor says, "It is entirely possible and likely that it doesn't matter what you do – your family probably won't step up. In fact, my family still hasn't gotten it more than fifteen years later! But after a lot of time and *a lot* of therapy, I realized that *I* could step up – that *I* could get it. My being miserable didn't make my family miserable, and it sure as hell wasn't making me happy. I learned to value myself and find other people to meet my needs that weren't met by my blood relatives. And I learned to meet a lot of those needs myself – giving myself that nurturance that I didn't get from my family."

Understanding the cause of one's eating disorder can sometimes be an important part of the recovery process inasmuch as uncovering the needs that are met through the eating disorder and learning to meet them in new, healthy ways is the key to a successful recovery. This deeper work of recovery usually must come after the initial period of crisis stabilization, in which a person decreases, and eventually stops, using eating disorder symptoms. Intensive therapy work cannot be done while a person is medically unstable due to an eating disorder – symptoms must be tackled before working on underlying issues: Waiting to understand the problem before fixing it can lead to a prolonged illness and decreased likelihood of recovery. Some elements of the eating disorder may not be understood for years, if ever. Put bluntly, a person can die waiting for the past to make sense. Eating disorder work must initially focus on the present moment.

There are different levels of treatment for eating disorders. Intensive outpatient treatment programs generally meet for a couple hours, three or so times per week. They tend to be "crash courses" in healthy living, also aiming to provide educative material about nutrition and breaking eating disorder patterns. Full day programs meet for several hours each day, at least five days per week. They involve different groups, covering topics such as nutrition, coping skills, medical issues, and relapse prevention. More intensive still are residential and inpatient treatment programs in which patients receive care on a twenty-four/seven basis. Residential programs tend to be longer term than inpatient programs and are completely voluntary, whereas inpatient programs are usually hospital-based and geared towards acute medical stabilization. There are also private outpatient doctors and therapists who work with clients struggling with eating disorders.

In most cases a number of these treatment levels are utilized to help a person achieve recovery. Treatment professionals recommend the least restrictive environment possible for recovery. Often a patient will be referred to a higher level of care if their current treatment setting is not having the desired effect, and it is recommended that patients "step down" from higher levels of care by joining intensive outpatient groups and meeting with private therapists, doctors, nutritionists, and psychiatrists. Tips for choosing an appropriate treatment team are discussed in Chapter 2.

When preparing to leave treatment or step down to a less structured level of treatment it is of utmost importance to establish a solid aftercare plan. According to Rebekah Bardwell Doweyko transitions are the strongest form of triggers because during times of foreign, new experiences, people automatically revert to patterns that are familiar and comfortable. If old, familiar patterns include eating disorder behaviors then that person must be on guard against possible relapse. Transitioning out of intensive treatment is among the first major tests of recovery. Coping skills such as honesty and using your voice can ease the way. When you have little slips – and everyone does – admit them. Talk about them.

"Find people who know how to help," says Rebekah. It's hard for anyone to be objective about their own behavior, and even more so for people fresh out of treatment for eating disorders. Rebekah cautions that "people left to their own devices will most likely assume wrong." It's not enough to simply find a treatment team, however. Your team will need to know how to best help you. Be open with them and speak up about what you need and don't need, what is helpful and what is not. Bear in mind, however, that if you are transitioning out of a more intensive form of treatment, such as residential or inpatient care, then you can expect some significant changes in therapy style. This will be addressed more fully in Chapter 2.

In the early stages of your recovery, you will likely find yourself missing treatment at times. This is neither harmful nor unhealthy, and it does not make you "sick" or "crazy." Knowing that this is a common occurrence among those leaving treatment provides you with an opportunity to make a solid aftercare plan.

Says Melanie Smith, once aftercare coordinator, now clinical program manager for the Renfrew Center, "After treatment, especially if you had a positive experience and are moving towards recovery, or experiencing recovery, periods of missing treatment are to be expected." Treatment is a time when you have people around you literally at all times who are nurturing and supportive and always there for you day or night. These are people who truly understand what you are going through and they have a certain empathy that is less-often found in the outside world. In treatment you have the support of experienced and knowledgeable professionals *and* you have the support of your peers – people with similar stories, experiences, and feelings whose paths have converged with yours. It's normal and natural to miss these things. However, the support and safety experienced in treatment should be taken as a sort of "preview of coming attractions." You can and should attempt to put a system in place in your home environment that will support you after you leave the confines of the treatment center or hospital.

"Building that support system before you get there is really important," says Melanie. "Know who those people are who you can go to when you are having a bad day. Let them know what you will need from them ahead of time, before you leave treatment." Melanie recounts that a recently-discharged patient in her mid forties who is divorced and has virtually no contact at all with her family still has a perfectly sustainable recovery. Her support system consists of her closest friends and neighbors. Melanie recommended that this woman start doing family therapy with her friends, since they are the ones closest to her in life and they are the ones who will support her. Rather than force a fabricated "support system" that is of no interest to both her family and herself, this woman identified her rocks – the ones who will be there for her in her times of need. The family therapy is needed to ensure that proper boundaries are in place so that both the woman and her friends receive adequate support and guidance and learn to support each other without harming themselves.

"That's what's really important," Melanie continues, "once you figure that out, it can work. The last thing you want to do is make a support system where the friends are being frustrated and not really getting anything out of it." Family therapy helps families – and any close support network – maintain healthy relationships and function within specific boundaries.

Perhaps the best way to ensure your own success after treatment is to develop a relapse-prevention plan, especially if recovery was not maintained following previous treatment experiences. In determining your relapse-prevention plan it is wise to work together with your therapist to brainstorm ways to deal with your specific anticipated challenges upon leaving treatment, including things that you struggle with in the present moment that may become more challenging as you step down from therapy.

❧ Aurora

The first time she went to treatment, Aurora felt forced into it by her family, her outpatient treatment team, and her school. She didn't want to be there and she fought the system tooth and nail, complying with neither the rules nor the treatment process. She did not take ownership of her own recovery and thus relapsed shortly after her discharge date.

When Aurora went back to treatment a couple of years later, things were different. For the first time she wanted recovery and she chose it for herself, taking responsibility for the process. She had a lot of guilt over her first time in treatment. She looked back at how she acted on her symptoms and argued needlessly with those trying to help her and considered what a wasted opportunity it had been, an opportunity that she was lucky to have had.

Knowing that few people with eating disorders have the option to go into intensive treatment, let alone go there twice, Aurora was determined to make her recovery stick this time. She accepted and believed that her team was there to help her and that they had her best interests at heart. She saw that they were going after her eating disorder, not after *her*.

Towards the end of her second residential stay, Aurora lost her father to a lengthy illness. He was the closest person to her in the world and at times her grief was unbearable. At first she felt numb and disconnected, much the way her eating disorder made her feel.

Soon it was time to leave treatment. Aurora worked with her therapists to develop an aftercare plan that would account not only for the fact that this would be her first time going home with a plan to keep up with her recovery, but also for the fact that maintaining her recovery in the face of such tremendous loss would be doubly hard. It was decided that she would stay with family for a month before returning home.

Surrounded by family, Aurora had a lot of healthy support. That was already different than what she had tried in the past: Avoiding family and isolating herself from those who cared. It was still difficult to open up and accept her family's support. She spent a lot of time running away from their guidance and empathy. While she was with her family she kept up with her outpatient team via phone sessions. When she returned home she got a job which provided structure until she was able to return to college. Aurora pushed herself to attend support groups and to connect with others who were further along in their recovery and could offer additional support.

Aurora learned that recovery is not a solitary activity, nor is it a spectator sport. A lot of times she felt like she had to do it on her own, but there are lots of avenues for support. There are friends, family, support groups, and twelve-step meetings. She was always a strong individual, but with the backing of her support system she was stronger and better able to weather her recovery journey despite tremendous and unexpected challenges.

"I always tried to do everything alone. I had to give that up. Surrender."

Part of planning an aftercare regimen is recognizing that while you cannot change everything around you, you *can* change how you react to your surroundings. If, for example, your family or friends are constantly on diets and talking about food or weight loss, it will be difficult – if not impossible – to change their behavior. You can, however, choose not to let it derail your recovery. Jodi Krumholz, director of nutrition for the Renfrew Center, tells clients, "You are not made of glass. You will not break if something triggering is said." It's not about what happens, it's about what you make of it. This likely requires the types of changes in your thinking and behavior that you worked on in treatment. Now the trick is going back to old situations with your new coping skills.

Jessica

When she was preparing to leave residential treatment for the second time, Jessica was to complete a relapse-prevention notebook given to her by her therapist. She struggled at first to go through the cheesy exercises and homework assignments. She hadn't done any of this the first time and she'd relapsed shortly after her discharge from treatment. She reasoned that she might as well give it a shot. What did she have to lose?

A sports enthusiast, Jessica turned her relapse prevention into a multi-faceted "game plan":

- Jessica took stock of her problem areas in which she was likely to struggle when she returned home from treatment.

- She accepted that her parents would probably not change their eating habits, which they had promised to do the first time Jessica was in treatment. The change hadn't even lasted one week. This time Jessica knew that nothing would be different in this department so she was going to have to come at the situation in a new way. Going home with the acceptance that her parents wouldn't change made Jessica stronger – she learned to go outside of her comfort zone to eat with them.

- She completed the relapse-prevention workbook given to her by her therapist. This project served to help Jessica set things in place while she was in a healthy mindset so that she could reference her coping skills later on during difficult moments. This would help her to avoid acting out of emotional pain.

- Jessica wrote a letter from her healthy self to her struggling self (see Chapter 7 for an example of one of these).

- She listened to the guidance of her treatment team and actually did as she was advised, something very difficult for Jessica who usually thought she knew best. The hardest piece of advice she received in treatment was that she should stop playing softball. The first time Jessica heard her team say this, she thought they "were crazy and had lost any sense they once had in some previous lifetime." It was never going to happen. Jessica loved softball and the first time she left treatment she refused to listen to them. She went home and started playing again, which sent her spiraling back into a full-blown relapse. When she was preparing to leave treatment for the second time and once again was advised to give up her place on the softball team, Jessica still found it difficult but she also saw that it was the healthier option to quit. She had to grieve the loss of her dream of being a star softball player, but Jessica believes that listening to her team about this issue has saved her recovery.

- Jessica recited positive affirmations over and over again, even though they seemed "childish and hokey." After some time, she came to believe them.

- She stopped making demeaning jokes about herself as a defense mechanism. She toned down her sarcasm, which she often hid behind, and instead Jessica faced her true feelings.

- Jessica talked about the really painful and private struggles she faced in her life. Things she'd never before said out loud because of the shame she felt and how hard those things were to say. She lowered her "perfect life" façade and allowed herself to be vulnerable.

- Finally, Jessica was willing to change – to hurt, to feel, to cry, to let go, to live, to be happy, and to stop judging herself in front of a mirror. She was ready to admit imperfection, to be honest and open, and to give up her identity as "the anorexic girl." She never thought she could give up that title, but once she did, she found she could live without it and that there was more to her than her eating disorder. Jessica was willing to grow.

Jessica's advice regarding relapse-prevention plans: "They may feel dumb at the time, but they work when you go home!"

Jessica went home knowing full well that motivation waxes and wanes. Sometimes, she knew, she would not be able to rely on her feelings, and would have to instead allow her thoughts to guide her. This is a great example of the "wise mind" model in dialectical behavior therapy (DBT) developed by Marsha Linehan.

According to the wise mind model there are two ways to make decisions – on your emotions or on your thoughts. Acting only on your emotions is termed "emotion mind" and acting only on your thoughts is called "reasonable mind." When you operate from emotion mind you may neglect certain facts. Cognitive distortions, such as black-and-white thinking or catastrophizing, may cloud your judgment. When you operate from "reasonable mind" you may neglect to consider your true feelings and desires. The optimal way to make decisions is to operate from "wise mind" which is a healthy balance between the two in which all components of the decision-making process are incorporated.

Upon stepping down from more intensive forms of treatment, and especially when coming home from residential or inpatient care, it can be easy to slip into "emotion mind." During these trying moments it is important to "factor in the facts." In other words, don't let your feelings completely run the show. Your thoughts are important, too.

A professor of mine at Florida Atlantic University, Dr. Paul Peluso, teaches aspiring counselors about the effect of emotions on memory. Everyone has memories that are positive, neutral, and negative. But our emotions can skew our memories. When we feel happy, we tend to skew the meaning of our memories toward the positive such that our positive memories are positive; some of our neutral memories are positive; and even some of our negative memories shift up toward the neutral range. When we feel sad, the opposite holds true. Our negative memories are negative; some of our neutral memories are negative; and even some of our positive memories shift toward the neutral or even negative range.

Our feelings lend an element of meaning to our memories. If such drastic changes can occur in our memories of things we've had the chance to think through many times, then just imagine the impact of strong emotions on our current reality! Factor in the facts. Take a step back and consider your options. Beware of letting feelings dictate actions and attitudes.

Something else to be on the lookout for is complacency – a sense that you are "cured." The perfect recovery is as much a myth as the perfect eating disorder. There is no such thing. Recovery from eating disordered thoughts by definition requires the shedding of cognitive distortions such as all-or-nothing thinking. My dad often reminds me, "Don't get too high; don't get too low." This means to say that extremes are dangerous.

Feeling too high is dangerous because it is unsustainable. Ultimately during such times I would soon come crashing down, because I'd gotten to a place where I thought things were so great and I would never feel sad or upset again. Getting too high is dangerous because it builds unrealistic expectations.

Getting too low, on the opposite side of the spectrum, does the same thing in a different way. Instead of thinking things will never be upsetting again, you can come to believe that things will never be good or even okay again. This is dangerous because it can lead to hopelessness and thoughts such as, "If things will never improve anyway, why bother trying?"

I try to stay away from extremes. I'm neither on top of the world where nothing can shake me, nor am I crushed beneath the world where nothing can save me.

It helps to remember that life is a constant ebb and flow of thoughts, emotions, and activities. According to a lesson I once had in dialectical behavior therapy (DBT), the highest intensity of any feeling lasts about eight seconds. Eight seconds! If you can stick it out through those eight seconds, it will get easier (so long as you truly *feel* it – no fighting and no prolonging). We are programmed, in a sense, to maintain equilibrium. What goes up must come down, but what goes too far down must also come back up. It's a balance and like anything else, it takes time and practice to achieve a level of confidence – in the process, in your recovery, and in yourself. Recovery, and life as a whole, is the process of becoming who you are. These kinds of things rarely take the form of a sudden revelation, but rather a slow, steady progression. You don't just jump to the top – you climb there one foot at a time.

"The thing about confidence," says Rebekah Bardwell Doweyko, "is that confidence comes in time. The only way to build confidence is to allow yourself to struggle [and] to not numb through the struggle." That is what leads to coming out on the other side with the ability to look back and say, "That was really hard, but I made it."

Chapter 2

Building and Using a Treatment Team

"Allowing yourself to fully trust in somebody…can be very healing."

– Rebekah Bardwell Doweyko

Building and using a professional support system is essential to the maintenance of recovery from eating disorders, particularly in the earlier stages of recovery and during struggles at any point. While you certainly have the ability to learn the tools and skills needed for a healthy, meaningful life, eating disorder recovery – much like treatment – is not something you should attempt on your own. In working with a treatment team you give yourself a much greater advantage as you fight your eating disorder. Think about it – the eating disorder is a formidable opponent with many tricks and deceptions up its sleeve. The more people you get on your side the more you increase your chances of success.

The most common team members working with those in recovery from eating disorders are therapists, medical doctors, nutritionists, and psychiatrists. If you are not familiar with the healthcare providers in your area, be sure to do your homework before going in to the office. You may also seek recommendations from a trusted practitioner or treatment center. Things to consider before scheduling your first appointment include:

- professional reputation of the practitioner

- matters of insurance

- matters of payment (some practitioners offer a sliding scale based on need)

- the expertise of the practitioner in areas pertinent to your case.

It is generally advisable to work with practitioners genuinely specializing in eating disorders. A crash course on eating disorder treatment does *not* make a true expert. Ideally you should look for someone with adequate training and experience in the field.

Therapists

Since you will be delving most deeply into your story with your therapist, it is imperative to find one who at the very least understands eating disorders. Ideally you should find a therapist whose ideas about eating disorders align with yours, or if your ideas are unclear, confused, or otherwise distorted, find a therapist whose approach to eating disorders feels right or whose ideas align with the ideas of someone you trust. *Remember that when you go for your initial interview with your therapist you are interviewing them just as much as they are interviewing you.*

According to Rebekah Bardwell Doweyko, if no eating disorder specialist is available in your area, working with a substance abuse or other addiction specialist is a reasonable alternative. Both disorders share common elements, such as all-or-nothing thinking and the need to develop healthy coping skills for recovery to be possible.

Trusting your therapist can take time. If you aren't comfortable sharing your deepest secrets on the first day, that is completely normal and even healthy. Just as any connection takes time to develop, so too does a therapeutic relationship. Before calling it quits and searching for a new therapist, it is recommended that you give your current arrangement a fair chance by attending at least a few sessions.

Melanie Smith, once aftercare coordinator, now clinical program manager for the Renfrew Center of Florida, cautions her clients not to decide too quickly that they don't click with their new therapist, especially after stepping down from an inpatient or residential setting.

"Transitioning from a therapist that you really trust – especially if you are ambivalent about leaving treatment – to a new therapist is very hard," she says. "It's hard for you to initially feel in the first couple of sessions that you *do* click because there is that either conscious or unconscious comparison of old therapist to new therapist." Melanie explains that because it will be a new relationship and a new start – and in a completely different setting (e.g. the difference between seeing an inpatient therapist almost every day versus seeing an outpatient therapist once or twice a week) – you need to have realistic expectations that the type and intensity of the new relationship will be wholeheartedly different.

Melanie emphasizes, "It is such a difference. In residential you are seeing your therapist individually. You are seeing them in groups. You are seeing them in the hallways, at meals, always… They really do know every bit and piece of your life at that moment in time, whereas your outpatient therapist only gets a snapshot once a week."

This fundamental difference means that it's unrealistic to expect your new outpatient therapist to read you as well as your residential therapist, at least initially. It means that you need to be more motivated to disclose more in order to help your new therapist understand you better. Melanie recommends sticking it out, even if it doesn't feel ideal, for at least a month or two: "Surprisingly, working through that resistance and talking about it is one of the most powerful ways to build a therapeutic relationship." Then, if you have truly given the therapeutic relationship a fair chance of success and you have stuck it out for a number of sessions and don't see any real improvements, it may be time to take a different approach.

℘ Taylor

Taylor was able to do a lot of important work with her treatment team, both around her recovery and around other real issues in her life, such as the loss and neglect she'd experienced and the disappointment over the fact that she would most likely never get what she wanted or needed from her surviving family members. After her mother's passing, Taylor's relationship with her father was virtually nonexistent, and her relationship with her brother was rocky as well. Fortunately Taylor found support in other places, most notably in her rabbi's family and in her treatment team.

Although her initial therapist helped her tremendously through the loss of her mother and the subsequent grieving process, there came a time when Taylor recognized that she needed to move on to a new therapist.

"Because I started seeing her before my mom got sick, everything became about my mother," says Taylor. "And because of that, I was able to see that I wasn't getting what

I needed from her anymore. I needed someone with a different perspective."

Taylor began seeing a new therapist, with whom she also did a lot of important work. But once again there came a point of stagnation. Taylor already recognized the signs of lack of continued progress, and after discussing it with her second therapist, she moved on to her third.

"There were many levels to my therapy, and each time I switched from one therapist to the next, it was like I moved up a level," Taylor explains. "…almost like the levels of a video game!" she jokingly adds.

While she recognizes that not everyone must switch to a new therapist during a new stage of life, Taylor feels that in her specific case it was necessary. She also switched psychiatrists at one point because of a lack of reliability. It took her a long time to finally make the switch, mostly because she loved her psychiatrist so much. But because the psychiatrist was so difficult to reach, didn't return phone calls, and had few openings for appointments, Taylor knew that she needed to find someone else to fill that spot on her treatment team.

"I needed to take care of myself," she says, "I deserve to have a psychiatrist who I can reach during an emergency. I am paying for those services and I ought to have reliable care."

And because of her work in therapy, Taylor was able to evaluate the situation without an all-or-nothing filter.

"I finally realized that no matter how much I liked her, I needed to find someone else who was more reliable and who could help in an emergency. I don't love or like her any less as a person, but I still can see that she is not able to fill that need for me anymore."

Just as in real life things aren't always perfect, so too in therapy you may find that aspects of the relationship are less than ideal. How can you improve the relationship with your therapist and develop a stronger rapport?

Says Rebekah Bardwell Doweyko, "First and foremost by being honest about it. Telling the therapist, 'I'm having a difficult time connecting. I'm not so sure what it is,' or, 'I know what it is.' Letting the therapist know what's helpful and what's not." Rebekah stresses that a therapist is working for you the same way that a lawyer is working for you or a doctor or a plumber. "Let them know what you want and what you need," she adds, "It's really important to be open and honest and to be open to [having this] discussion."

Often it is the relationships that are rocky at the outset, that eventually grow to be warm, nurturing, and the most advantageous. Though it takes time, it is ultimately an investment in building and maintaining a solid foundation for your continued recovery.

"Allowing yourself to fully trust in somebody, to surrender, to believe that they may know better than you do when it comes to your health and your eating disorder or addiction – or whatever it is that you're struggling with – and just having somebody that you can trust and let take care of you can be very healing," says Rebekah. There is often a sense of relief after a first therapy session, particularly for someone who is engaging in the therapeutic process for the first time. Even though first sessions are rarely concerned with intensive work, the empathy and support of the therapist combined with identifying challenges and setting goals, inspires hope for many people. You may find that sharing your struggles and being met with a listening ear is comforting and even encouraging.

A therapy session is a microcosm of real life. The thoughts and feelings, behaviors and boundaries that you practice and experience in sessions (and between sessions) can all be taken into your everyday life. You may be aware of some common "therapeutic boundaries" that give order to the client–therapist relationship. This is precisely why those rules are in place.

Rebekah explains, "A lot of times, because of the eating disorder or other addictions, families don't set as many limits as they should – or their limits were too harsh. And so there's a lack of [healthy] boundaries that exists. The therapist can be the person who actually sets up boundaries and becomes a role model – somebody who models healthy coping skills and boundaries."

Medical doctors

It is to your benefit to find a primary care physician knowledgeable about eating disorders, if at all possible. A competent eating disorder specialist will be more adept at uncovering symptoms and identifying physical illness caused by an eating disorder as such. The physical examination should include specific tests such as measuring the difference in pulse and blood pressure between lying down, sitting, and standing positions. If the numbers are significantly different, then it is possible that the heart is being made to work harder than it should. There are a multitude of other tests that may be required depending on your specific condition. Possible tests include electrocardiogram, blood tests, and bone density scans.

A good primary care doctor should ideally collaborate with the rest of your treatment team in order to fill in the medical piece of the puzzle. This will help you and your team make informed decisions about things like exercise. Although this is not entirely a medical decision, it *is* an important factor. You will most likely be asked to sign information release forms before team members can communicate with each other about your case.

In my personal case, my doctor was my key lifeline throughout my early recovery. Initially I saw her every week, then once every other week, and then we eventually tapered down to once every few months. She was warm and kind and was the first person who I felt really "got me" about the eating disorder. She remained among my strongest allies against my eating disorder throughout my treatment in the hospital, day treatment, and finally residential treatment. In fact, she was instrumental in helping me get into treatment in the first place. Shortly before I was referred to residential treatment, I described my idea of a decent lunch: Cottage cheese squished between the two end pieces of a loaf of bread. My doctor made a face and told me, "I'm five months pregnant and crave weird foods, but I just lost my appetite. You're going to Renfrew."

Nutritionists

A nutritionist should be able to offer not only educative information, but also support and encouragement as you venture out of your comfort zone and into more advanced stages of recovery. Upon finding a qualified nutritionist specializing in the treatment of eating disorders, you will probably be given several tasks in addition to nutritional guidance. Among the most common are specific food lists, meal planning, and food journals.

Specific food lists aim to heighten your awareness of specific problem areas concerning the food-related elements of your eating disorder. Types of food lists might include lists of foods you avoid or are afraid to eat (fear foods), foods you purge, and foods you binge on or overeat on a regular basis. Through making these lists you may discover certain patterns and become more cognizant of your choice to institute new patterns.

Meal planning is helpful especially in the beginning of recovery when internal senses of hunger, fullness, and intuition regarding food choices are unreliable. The idea is that by making detailed lists of specific foods, you will be better able to meet your nutritional goals in an efficient manner than if you were to attempt to make intuitive choices when your signals are off base.

Food journals are multi-faceted accounts of daily intake. First, they detail what foods you actually ate on a given day, as well as the amounts of each food. Typically calorie counting is avoided and, if need be, replaced by healthier methods of ascertaining quantities consumed, such as the exchange system. In the exchange system foods are divided into nutritional categories based on grams of each nutrient they contain. Each nutrient has a set number of grams that constitutes an "exchange." For example, seven grams of protein make up one protein exchange. The food journals also include levels of hunger and satiety as well as your thoughts and feelings about each meal and snack. Obviously the effectiveness of the food journal method will depend upon your effort to share the full story.

Your nutritionist will likely ask you to bring in your recent food journals to each appointment where the two of you will review them together. In addition to providing a certain sense of accountability, the food journals help you express yourself in a systematic – and possibly more comfortable – way, and provide information which will help your nutritionist target new areas to work on with you while providing the necessary support.

Aurora

Aurora considers food journals to be an instrumental part of her recovery, especially during times when she needs a bit more structure and support around food and eating. During a struggle she is more likely to gloss over issues of restriction, binging, and other symptoms. The food journals force her to closely examine how she is really doing food-wise and help to ensure accountability.

"They help me see if I am missing anything that I need to be eating or if the times are okay, if I'm eating frequently enough, etc. I also like doing them because they bring up things like food choices and my ability to share my food choices."

Like a lot of people battling eating disorders, Aurora initially struggled to overcome food-related shame and embarrassment. She worried about what other people would think about her because of what she was eating, or how much she was eating, or how little. Sometimes it was even hard for her to share her thoughts and feelings with her treatment team. The food journals helped her overcome a lot of this difficulty.

"I journal a lot on my food journals about feelings that come up. They're called 'journals' for a reason." She writes about her hunger and fullness, where she was when she ate, what was going on around her, how her body image was, what her mood was. If she just got into an argument that was still causing her distress, that could impact her eating and so she includes it on her food journal. She also uses her food journals to express her individuality.

"I like to personalize them," she says. "The artist in me likes to color code them and make them all pretty."

Psychiatrists and other forms of support

In choosing a psychiatrist it is crucial to consider the doctor's areas of expertise and specialty. Every medication has side effects and some may be more pronounced in or hazardous to an individual with a history of an eating disorder. A qualified psychiatrist should recognize these dangers and treat accordingly.

Something else to consider is joining a support group or working a twelve-step program. A particularly helpful fellowship is Eating Disorders Anonymous (EDA). Alcoholics Anonymous (AA) is also helpful for many who struggle with eating disorders because of the themes and challenges that underlie both eating disorders and alcoholism. Rebekah Bardwell Doweyko cautions, however, that in "AA you want to tread lightly because some AA meetings talk about restricting wheat and flour." She also stresses the positive aspects of these groups. "People can go to AA and just substitute the word 'alcohol' for their eating disorder and it's the same. And there are AA meetings found everywhere. They even have them on cruise ships. So let's say you're on a cruise and you had a hard time with your meal. Maybe you are triggered by the abundance of food at the buffets – you can go to an AA meeting and substitute 'alcohol' for 'food' and it can be very helpful."

In order to recover, you must be true to yourself and ask the really difficult questions, no matter how scary they seem.

- What *is* life in recovery?

- Who am I without my eating disorder?

- What keeps me stuck? (i.e. what do I get out of having an eating disorder that I'm afraid to give up?)

- What will it be like to take care of myself?

- How am I *really* doing?

This last question is especially important. In order to maintain your recovery you *must* be able to accept the ups and downs of the process. Everyone has bad days. Even people who have been in recovery for many years occasionally have setbacks or slips or challenging thoughts and feelings. Having the acceptance that *this is where you are right now* breaks through the layers of denial and rationalization. It aids in your ability to stick out the tough times without falling into the trap of all-or-nothing. Maybe in the moment after a slip you're not doing terrific, but you're not doing terrible either. In short, acceptance helps you be real.

What happens if you slip really far back? What if you truly are in danger of a relapse, or maybe you already have relapsed? Take a deep breath. All is not lost. It may be a difficult road back, but you can make it. Be honest with your team, or, if you haven't seen your team in a while, get back in touch. Be upfront about your struggles. Remember, they've heard it all and they will be able to help you put things into perspective. A slip doesn't equal a relapse and a relapse doesn't equal a failure. There's no shame in having a problem – it's what you do about it that matters.

Jessica

Towards the end of her first time in residential treatment, Jessica's psychiatrist met with her to discuss her progress and chances of maintaining recovery after her discharge date. Jessica had been non-compliant with the rules for the past several days and was acting out in every way possible. Punching walls, holding onto food rituals and other eating disorder symptoms. A storm raged inside Jessica. She was jealous of everyone, it seemed. She wanted others' looks, clothing sizes, families, stories, personality… Instead of working through her thoughts and feelings, Jessica acted out. The consequences that ensued did little to help her get back on track.

At a certain point just prior to her discharge, Jessica gave up. She knew she needed treatment, but it was the one thing she just didn't excel at, so why bother trying? She'd been in treatment for over five weeks but still didn't think she was "sick enough" to be there. She wanted to be sick enough. She wanted to deserve help. She wanted to be good at this recovery thing, but she just *wasn't*!

Her psychiatrist sat her down and discussed her struggles with her. The meeting ended with him telling her that he would see her again soon. Jessica knew he was right, but she was unfazed. Then he said, "Everyone has a different road to recovery. Yours may have a break because you aren't ready for this kind of treatment yet. Your road has different bumps from anyone else's. Your recovery goes at your pace, not ours."

That message carried Jessica through until a few months later when she was readmitted to the same facility. This time she was ready. She went in knowing that "this is it." She knew it would be hard but didn't know *how* hard until she broke down in one of her first group therapy sessions. She burst into tears, sobbing her heart out, feeling unworthy of living. She went into crisis mode and in that moment became suicidal. She recounts that it was the scariest feeling of her life.

The therapist who ran the group talked to her afterwards for a half hour. She listened to Jessica and put her arms around her and conveyed through her actions and tone of voice that she cared about Jessica. Nevertheless, the next day Jessica's team moved her down a level in the program, thus revoking, at least temporarily, certain privileges. Frustrated and ready to storm out of treatment, Jessica packed her bags and signed a seventy-two hour notice letting her team know she intended to leave.

Her treatment team called her to an emergency meeting to discuss her intention to leave the program against medical advice. They were much tougher on Jessica this time than they were the first time around. They were firm but caring and eventually persuaded Jessica that they were only trying to help her. The team leader looked Jessica in the eyes and said, "The ways we tried to help you during your first stay with us obviously didn't work. We failed you."

Jessica was crushed and felt guilty. *My team didn't fail me*, she thought, *I failed them.* It was the other way around! She looked at her therapist, the same one she'd worked with the first time. She respected her therapist and felt a strong bond with her. Jessica didn't want to fail her. While she didn't like or agree with everything her team did, she understood that they were ultimately on the same team. The Get-Jessica-Well team. She understood their strictness to a certain extent and realized that nothing in her life would change for the better unless she was honest with her team. That was the only way to get anything real out of this program.

Opening up to her team for the first time, Jessica turned over her cell phone which she was not permitted to have with her in treatment. She also told on herself for breaking several other rules. There were consequences, and Jessica knew there would be. But even though it was unpleasant, Jessica continued to literally force herself to be honest with her team and give up the secrets that kept her sick.

Despite her poor track record at the center, Jessica succeeded in convincing her nutritionist that she should be permitted a certain mealtime privilege. She wrote a letter detailing why she felt she deserved it – her hard work, her struggles to be open and real, and her willingness to finally work with her treatment team. Jessica's nutritionist responded by telling her that in all honesty she had not been planning to award that privilege to Jessica at this time, but that Jessica's letter was an impressive display of owning the process of recovery. She told Jessica that she would allow her the privilege she requested, on a trial basis. If there was even one mealtime slip up, the privilege would be revoked. Jessica agreed and made good on her word. It was extremely uncomfortable at times to follow through, but Jessica pushed herself. She was not a quitter. Making that deal with her nutritionist solidified in Jessica's mind the idea of working together with her nutritionist, therapist, psychiatrist, and doctors. She was truly a part of her team. In time, Jessica's bond with her treatment team grew stronger and they were able to work together towards the day when Jessica would discharge from the facility and be told, "You made it. We're proud of you. And we hope to never see you here again!"

Although many of the individuals whose stories appear within this book have reached recovery after undergoing treatment at the inpatient level of care, it should be noted that this is not the case for everyone. Inpatient/residential treatment is not the only way to recovery and it, in itself, does not guarantee recovery. Andrew, for example, recovered at the outpatient level of care at the Marino Therapy Centre in Ireland after an unsuccessful stay in an inpatient hospital setting.

Andrew

Andrew left the hospital disappointed. He had wanted help, truly wanted it. But the hospital at which he found himself was unable to offer him help in the way he needed it. Sure, it was structured. But perhaps *too* structured. There were rules and regulations and restrictions, and relatively no personal attention.

"I went in in good faith," says Andrew, "but they took away my power. They gave me a set of rules. To me, recovery is being completely free from food [obsessions] and being able to live a normal life. The hospital program was focused on maintaining a healthy body weight. There was no one-to-one counseling. To me, it was a joke and soon afterwards I was back to where I started."

Thankfully Andrew found the Marino Therapy Centre.

"The Centre had its own approach," he says. At the Marino Therapy Centre Andrew was encouraged by an extensive support network. He was provided with one-to-one counseling, group therapy, and plenty of opportunities to discuss his process and progress. It was exactly what Andrew needed – to be heard, to be understood. Whereas other treatments felt like a professional trying to cure a patient, treatment at the Centre had a much more personal approach. It wasn't focused exclusively on behaviors or weight, and it treated each man and woman as an individual with a unique story and unique needs.

"That's why the hospital failed for me," says Andrew. "We were always told about barriers and boundaries and limitations. It didn't make sense to me. If recovery is possible then you shouldn't need limitations – you should be free to make healthy choices for yourself."

"People are screaming for hospital beds," Andrew laments, "there aren't enough beds for clients with eating disorders." Andrew recovered at a clinic that takes on as clients many individuals who have been previously hospitalized. Those same clients often gain more in their recoveries at the outpatient level of care than they did in the hospital. Andrew concludes that "it's not beds that you need – it's people with the right skills to treat the problem."

"They call the shots," Andrew says, explaining that the Marino Therapy Centre staff do not play around. "They tell it like it is," he says, "they gave me back the power to change my own life."

Chapter 3

CELEBRATING YOUR TRUE SELF

"The way to build self-esteem is
by doing estimable acts."

— Rebekah Bardwell Doweyko

Who are you?

When you hear this question, what answers come to mind? Are
you a son or daughter? Sibling? Parent? Friend? Are you a student
or employee? What about member of a sports team or other
recreational or professional group? You are probably several of
these and more. Throughout your life you fill many different roles.
Some roles are transient parts of your development, stages you
pass through along the way. Some are more permanent elements
of your identity. Some roles are healthy and others are not.

Eating disorder patient. This is not the most objectively
healthy role, but a lot of people meet certain needs through it.
Eating disorders are many things to many people. They can be
a form of communication or control, a way to numb painful
feelings, and in many cases a sense of identity. It is very common
for individuals in recovery from eating disorders to struggle with
their identities, especially if their eating disorders have consumed
their lives for a significant period of time. An unhealthy sense of
identity can serve as a barrier to recovery.

ℰ𝒾 Jessica

Growing up, Jessica was very self-confident. She was comfortable with her abilities in virtually everything she did up until she was sixteen. Her one area of self-consciousness was her body. She remembers that at one point as a young pre-teen her jeans size matched her age. Jessica's brother made cruel jokes about it, saying he would hate to see her when she was thirty.

Hearing mean comments so frequently from family members about her size and appearance led Jessica to believe she would someday need a tractor to get her out of bed. While this was far from the truth, Jessica was terrified of losing control over her body. In later years Jessica recognized that her brother most probably made mean, teasing jokes about her out of jealousy – Jessica performed better at school and in sports and therefore got more attention from their family and from teachers – but the comments still hurt.

She felt she had to control her body dimensions not only for the sake of her appearance but also for the sake of her identity. During her first year of college Jessica played on the girls' softball team on which the vast majority of the players were both physically large (muscular) and homosexual. Jessica made a connection between the two and assumed that if she was large then people would assume she was also homosexual. This exacerbated Jessica's fears of being a "big girl" and she began intentionally losing weight.

Soon Jessica's ego was bolstered by comments made by others about her shrinking body – comments like "I wish I had your willpower!" As her weight loss continued, Jessica began to develop "rules" about her appearance. She had to make sure certain bones were visible every time she looked in the mirror. This gave Jessica reassurance that she wasn't "too big." Because after all, being "too big" was not just about size – to Jessica it was about peer acceptance, sexuality, and self-worth.

"Many patients will come into treatment scared of losing the gains of the eating disorder," says Carolina Gaviria, Columbian psychologist and Renfrew aftercare coordinator. She goes on to explain that eating disorders can serve as a form of pseudo-protection against the tensions associated with growth into new stages of life. "Especially adolescence… growing up, paying bills, grocery shopping…" Change is often frightening. Carolina gently helps her clients understand that they don't need to use the eating disorder to escape the fear. "[You] are not alone. You have other people in your life who can guide you through the process. Other people go through the same thing. You don't have to do it alone. Yes, it's overwhelming and you probably will feel overwhelmed at first – and then it will become familiar… going through moments of anxiety and stress – you can get through it."

Carolina suggests that being true to oneself is a key factor in recovery. This goes beyond identifying things you like and don't like. It's about more than who-are-you, what-do-you-want, and where-are-you-going. What stage of development are you in and what does it mean to you? Being true to yourself is about who you are on the deepest, multi-faceted levels. It's about your core beliefs and identity.

 ## Andrew

It was horrible to be a man with an eating disorder, Andrew remembers. Throughout his struggle to overcome anorexia, Andrew encountered a multitude of stereotypes not only about his illness but also about his gender.

"First of all," Andrew states, "there is an expectation of men to stand on their own two feet." He says that feeling this pressure from society tempted him to "suffer in silence." He was afraid to seek treatment for what was commonly perceived as a woman's problem. Andrew felt the need to be a rock, bottle his emotions, and deal with problems in a "manly" way.

"I felt lonely and isolated," says Andrew of his eating disordered years. "I felt a bit like a freak, to be honest."

After nearly ten years of suffering, Andrew finally overcame his eating disorder with the help of an outpatient treatment centre in Ireland where he is from. He had to confront those stereotypes which haunted him and ultimately learn to express himself. He could still be strong for his family, but he didn't need to be an unfeeling "rock."

"I've become a new person," says a recovered Andrew. "I had to let go of who I was when I had an eating disorder and become a new person."

What is your identity? What is your gender identity, professional identity, sexual identity, spiritual identity?

What is your cultural identity?

"It's important, when you are determining your identity separate from your eating disorder, to explore your culture," says Carolina. She elaborates that culture is a multidimensional phenomenon. You probably belong to several different cultures, whether or not you are aware of it. Carolina explains that even within a specific setting, such as the Renfrew Center where she works, there are several different subgroups, each with its own form of group identity – on a basic level there are the patients and the staff members. Delving deeper there are groups within these groups. Patients might subgroup into age brackets or associate with those with whom they share similar religious values or career goals. Staff members may subgroup and identify as "therapists" or "students." They may work on the clinical side with patients, or in an office away from the patients. They may identify with one or more of these groups. It goes back to the roles mentioned in the opening of this chapter.

And those types of groups, I believe, are secondary to your true identity. Being a patient in a treatment center (or a therapist) is who you are in one setting. In another setting you may classify yourself as a family member or friend or teammate. You may be of a certain nationality, ethnic group, and religion. All of these factors – to a greater or lesser extent – make up your individual culture and, to a large extent, who you are on a consistent, permanent basis.

Your culture may influence your development of an eating disorder as well as how you go about recovery. Carolina shares that in Columbia the field of eating disorders treatment is only just beginning to develop, despite a long history of disordered eating and body image preoccupation in the country.

"In Columbia there are lots of plastic surgeons and lots of young women go to them for boob jobs, liposuction... the culture of the body is very marked," says Carolina. "There's the other side, too," she further states, "the food they eat is not very balanced. [There are] a lot of starches, fried foods..." This, she believes, has to do with the food grown in the country, such as sugar and grains. A typical meal in Columbia might consist of rice, beans, fried eggs, thick fried bacon, and fried plantains.

Aside from the issues of food and plastic surgery is the pressure to put forth a certain image and the stigma attached to having a problem such as an eating disorder. "There's a lot of social pressure to project a beautiful, nice, thin, friendly image... 'I know how to dance, study, be the perfect woman,'" says Carolina. She explains that it is difficult for many people to deal with the incongruence of the culture and feeling pressured to project an image that is not who you are. There is a lot of pretending. And if there is a problem, it is rarely if ever disclosed. "Columbia is a country of secrets," Carolina says. "We don't talk about those things." Rarely, in Columbia, does a family admit that a child or adolescent of theirs in struggling with such things. And if they do, they are reluctant to seek counseling for the whole family instead of just for that child. It has been this way for generations.

"Now it is starting to improve," says Carolina on a brighter note. "In terms of eating disorders, we have a couple of residential facilities." She admits that they are pretty basic, but a necessary first step in improving the situation for those in Columbia suffering from eating disorders.

The picture Carolina painted of the dominant culture of Columbia as she experienced it is a tribute to the complexities of both personal identity and the recovery process. I once met a woman who was struggling to maintain her commitment to Orthodox Judaism while in treatment. She told me it was crucial for her to keep kosher and observe the Sabbath and keep Jewish law to the best of her ability given the circumstances, because that is what defined her. She told me, "This is who I am. My Judaism is my identity. If I give it up, then who am I and what am I recovering for?"

A powerful message.

By the same token, you should be careful to ensure that elements of your identity do not become your *whole* identity.

Taylor

Taylor worked hard in recovery with the goal of holding a steady job. Once she achieved that, however, she attached herself a bit too strongly to her job title ("contractor") and thus was less able to differentiate between who she was at work and who she was as a person. In a sense it was similar to the way she previously identified with her eating disorder. If she didn't have her job, then who was she?

"Even today I don't fully know who I am," Taylor admits, "but I'm working on it." Taylor works on it by opening herself to new experiences. She tries new things and figures out not only what things make her happy, but also *why* they make her happy.

"Yesterday I was very depressed about something that happened at work," she says, "I hated my job and didn't know what to do. I was miserable. I wound up calling a friend and venting to her about the situation, which then turned into a friendly catching-up conversation."

Taylor also went through old journal entries and poems and other writings she's completed over the years.

"Today I realized that writing makes me incredibly happy. What I specifically choose to write about at any given moment really depends on my mood, but it's nice and enlightening to find and reread writings of mine from ten years ago. I like writing humor, I *love* writing songs. Sometimes I write somber pieces. The serious writing doesn't necessarily make me happy per se, but it gives me a better sense of who I am. And writing both, as different occasions arise, gives balance to my life."

It is of utmost importance for therapists and other treatment professionals to understand their clients on a deeper level than "eating disorder patient" and it is of even *greater* importance for the clients to understand *themselves* on a deeper level. Carolina Gaviria cautions that there are always feelings and beliefs around your culture. For example, "people may feel they are going against God's will if they speak against their culture, religion, etc." People tend to be protective of their cultures and fear giving their group a bad name. In treatment this fear can have detrimental effects, especially if something in the culture – as in

Carolina's example about Columbia – contributed to the illness or prevented prior recovery. This fear is often compounded by fears of stigma or stereotypes associated with different groups. For example, if someone is living with a disability, that person may be sensitive to stereotypes about laziness and living off the government. It's important for therapists to help encourage their clients to explore these thoughts, feelings, and beliefs in an open, nonjudgmental way. They must build empathy and trust with each client so that there is a safe space to share such information. For your part as a client, it is important to recognize areas that need further exploration and to allow yourself the possibility of self-discovery and acceptance.

Acceptance of *all* of your thoughts and feelings leads directly to acceptance of self. This is not to say that all thoughts are healthy, positive, and good. Many thoughts must be challenged and ultimately replaced by new, more balanced thoughts. But until you *accept* that you have those negative thoughts in the first place, you cannot hope to correct them. A bad thought doesn't make you a bad person.

Says Rebekah Bardwell Doweyko, "You can get in a fight with somebody and think, 'I want to stab them in the eye with this pen,' but you don't *do* it." She explains that the important thing is not to be afraid of your negative thoughts. Accept that you *have* them and maintain an awareness that you do not need to *act* on them. We all have irrational thoughts. It's just part of being human. "You can challenge your thought and really look at what evidence supports it and what evidence does not, and come up with a balanced thought."

Feelings help us navigate life. On any given day we experience a myriad of feelings – happy, sad, excited, nostalgic, angry, jealous... Just like our thoughts, our feelings help us by giving us valuable information about our world. They give us a roadmap of sorts. Sometimes our feelings are a bit off-kilter but within a range that is okay too. Everyone has bad days and good days. Some feelings are more pleasant than others, but *no feelings can hurt you.* Even intense feelings of sadness, loss, and shame. A professor of mine tells her clients that happy and sad are equally valid emotions. Crying and laughing are equally expressive and equally okay. You may not like everything you feel, and sometimes you may need to make adjustments by working in therapy. But just like your thoughts, you cannot heal your emotions without first accepting them. In time, your acceptance of all of your thoughts and feelings will lead to a fuller, deeper understanding and acceptance of self.

When you begin to discover, accept, and appreciate your true self – with all your intricacies and complexities – you begin to break your alliance with your eating disorder. No longer do the eating disorder's "rules" control your life. No longer is there that competition to be the "sickest." Why? Because the illness no longer defines you. Your name is not "Sick." Your name is _____ (fill in the blank).

Jessica

Jessica wasn't even aware of her competitiveness, but through her behaviors she unconsciously vied to be the sickest, the best at her eating disorder. A woman in treatment with Jessica brought this struggle to her attention after Jessica expressed frustration with her weight in comparison to others'. She didn't feel "sick enough."

"Jessica," the woman gently said, "You didn't see yourself when you first entered treatment. It didn't matter how much or how little you weighed. You may not have been the thinnest or the most physically ill, but the expression on your face was more hopeless than most who have walked through those doors."

For the first time, Jessica realized that the number on the scale had little to do with her health or sickness. The woman's comment also made Jessica aware of her desire to be sicker than everyone else and Jessica began to notice her tendency toward competition.

At lunch that day Jessica ate with only one other patient. The other patient had a much larger meal than Jessica had, yet Jessica engaged in an unspoken contest to finish her meal last. A therapist commented on Jessica's use of food rituals and Jessica recognized that she was using them in order to slow her eating and win the "contest." This insight did not sit well with her and she resolved to overcome her competition to be the sickest.

Over the course of her treatment, Jessica explored several core aspects of her personality and belief system. She pinpointed those things that are important to her – her spirituality and religious faith, her family, her puppies, sports. Friends. Friends are very important to Jessica. In her first town she was so popular and had so many acquaintances but, as she puts it, "Everything was just for show." She was idolized for being the younger sister of a popular football player at the high school. She was known as "Danny's Little Sister," not as Jessica. This, in fact, played into her identity struggles. After her family moved to a new town, Jessica had no friends. She was the unpopular new kid. Being "Danny's Little Sister" didn't earn her any points at her new school, especially after Danny graduated. Who was Jessica on her own? How would she be known?

For a while she was known as the "girl with an eating disorder," but this was not who Jessica truly was. She continued searching for those things that mattered to her. Perseverance and follow-through. If Jessica did something, she gave it her all. She never backed down for fear of failure.

There was no doubt in Jessica's mind that she excelled in this area. No way was Jessica a quitter.

Jessica finally determined the three things that she always wants present in her life: Drive. Determination. Desire. Those characteristics are at the core of Jessica's being. That is who she is. And *that* is how she wants to be known.

Know who you are. Not simply "Am I an athlete, a student, an employee…?" Those things are externals. What happens if they go away? Who are you then? What happens if you can no longer play sports or you finish school or you switch jobs? If you place too much importance on the external roles in your life, then you risk losing sight of your true self. Jessica is very much an athlete and a student, but she defines her essence as "Drive. Determination. Desire." Those are the things at her core that make her who she is. Her values and strengths make up her true self, just as your values and strengths make up your true self. It is so important to know who you are.

The very first therapy group that I co-facilitated with one of my professors was called "Discover Your Strengths." After completing a course taught by this instructor, I was invited to her private practice to help her run groups with her clients who were all recovering from addictions. The mindset of addiction and eating disorders are very similar, and since I am in recovery from an eating disorder I was able to draw from my knowledge and experience. We designed the group based on a fundamental belief of counseling – everyone has strengths. The challenge sometimes is employing your strengths in areas of your life that you are not accustomed to using them. The group was very hands-on and experiential. Group members used art, music, movement, and sound to help them identify and fortify their strengths. In one of our first sessions, we presented the group members with boxes of crayons. They were to introduce themselves by way of selecting three or four crayons and explaining their significance in as few words as possible.

The exercise was meant as a simple activity to get everyone in the mindset of thinking more abstractly, but what ensued was nothing less than spectacular. As the group unfolded, the crayons became the embodiment of our clients' strengths. One woman chose a crayon called "razzle-dazzle pink" because it represented her friendly, confident, and exuberant personality. Other crayons signified emotional stability, connection with others, and perseverance.

After the crayons had been chosen we asked our group members if they could take a crayon (strength) from any other person in the group, which one would they take and why. (There was a clamoring rush for "razzle-dazzle pink!") They then shared with each other what their new crayon represented to them and how they admired the strengths they saw in each other.

Just like any therapy group, these individuals became a microcosm of the "outside world." They had helped each other in sessions many times before, bouncing ideas around and building on each other's strengths, and today they developed a greater understanding of *how* they were able to do this – they were individuals but also part of a group. Each one brought their own special strengths into the room and, together, they created magic.

What are your skills? What are your strengths? At what do you excel? How can you use your talents to live a happy, fulfilling life, connect with others, and achieve your goals?

What are your dreams? What is the motivating force in your life? What do you *live for*? The importance of dreams cannot be stressed enough. A commitment to recovery is a commitment to life. Jen Nardozzi, National Training Manager of the Renfrew Center, asks her clients to determine their specific commitments in life, their specific dreams. "You need something bigger than yourself that is going to get you out of bed everyday," she says. This is true for anyone. Without passion, goals, and commitment, life is a monotonous string of events, chores, and errands. It's not enough to simply "love life" or "cherish family." These are vague ideas. As we will explore in Chapter 7, motivating dreams must be specific. What do you want to accomplish? Seriously think about it. If you could be anyone, do anything, go anywhere, who would you be, what would you do, where would you go? Sometimes it helps to reconnect with your childhood dreams. As we progress into adulthood, and especially if an eating disorder is involved, we lose a lot of the magic of imagination. It's lost but not *gone*. It's always still *there* – we just have to learn to tap into it again. Says Jen, "When you're a kid you let yourself imagine everything." Ask yourself what your life is *for*. Think *outside* the box and find something that overshadows your eating disorder. Something that motivates you to truly live, to love yourself and to love life. (These things are rarely found *inside* the box.)

 ## Aurora

"Create who you are." That was Aurora's motto and it was how she lived her life right up until tragedy and her eating disorder put it all on an indefinite hold. The periods in which she could not or would not express herself creatively were the darkest times of Aurora's life, and there were moments when she didn't even recognize herself. Getting back in touch with her creativity reminded her of who she truly was.

When Aurora was a young child she loved reading and being read to. She loved arts and crafts. Later on, when she learned to write, she loved that too and from then on she knew she would be a writer and an artist. She wrote and illustrated stories and showed them to her dad who always responded in warm, loving praise. This propelled Aurora to new heights, further developing her artistic talents. She experimented with drawing, poetry, graphic design, and photography. Creative endeavors were her forte.

When Aurora lost her father and brother, both at a young age, she felt a part of herself go with them. She lost touch with her creative passions which connected her with her true self. She felt almost unreal, walking around as though in a daze, utterly lost without the two greatest men in her life.

It wasn't until she joined an art therapy group in treatment that she began to create once more. At first it was tedious and difficult. A dance to which she had to relearn the steps. But she persevered and tapped into her imagination again and again, going deeper and deeper with each new project, until she was really using her creativity to express herself. The themes of her new work weren't always positive or happy – in fact most of her projects during this delicate time period were dark and even a bit frightful. But they were real and Aurora was found.

"Dark isn't necessarily bad" became Aurora's permission to herself to engage in new projects. She thought that if what she wrote or drew was dark and held negative messages, then people wouldn't want to read it or look at it. It was hard for her to accept the beauty in all stages of recovery, and really, in all stages of *life*. Especially when she is her true, honest self.

Standing in her own talent, her own strength, her own power, Aurora caught a glimpse of the woman she once was and she saw that she still *was* that woman. There was still a long road ahead but now she was back on it. Regaining her creativity was like fixing her car in preparation for the long journey ahead. Now she was driving down the road, picking up speed. As she ventures towards full recovery, Aurora leaves a trail of poetry, drawings, and collages. Some happy, others sad, but all real and passionate.

"My passion is what makes me *me*," she says. "Everyone has something that they love, something that they are passionate about. I know that if I follow my passion, that if I trust it… it will take me in the right direction."

The bulk of "following your passion" comes *after* a healthy routine is established. Rebekah Bardwell Doweyko warns that sitting around the house in your pajamas all day, not practicing proper hygiene, and acting in ways contrary to your core values *will lower your self-esteem.* "The way to build self-esteem is by doing estimable acts," she says. "It's an estimable act to get up in the morning and go to work and be productive." Rebekah states that *productivity is the best way to combat depression.*

The challenge lies in the lethargy and lack of motivation inherent in depression. When you feel depressed and apathetic, it can be hard to get going. But ceasing to be productive only exacerbates the depression, and in turn, the lack of productivity. When you find yourself caught in this vicious cycle, that's when you turn to your dreams and passions. Rebekah advises, "Examine other talents and desires, have recreational interests and social interests. Put yourself out there. Take risks. Make new discoveries."

Korrie

A reputation is a hard thing to change. Korrie discovered this fairly early in life after realizing, partway through high school, that her reputation left much to be desired. Her friends were few and her teachers were constantly frustrated with her lack of attendance and her sense of entitlement.

Korrie did things *her* way. It was her way or no way at all. No one could make her follow the rules. There was nothing helpful in the rules for Korrie, anyway. If she had a headache because of her eating disorder then that meant she was "sick" and "special" and deserved to leave school. Korrie did what she felt she was entitled to do. She was above the rules, humoring them at times only for her own benefit.

Then one day everything changed. Korrie looked around and saw that in school she had no one. No allies. No friends. No mentors. She had alienated herself from every possible source of support. Previously, no one could have dreamed of getting Korrie to admit fault – not for anything! But in this moment, Korrie looked at herself under a magnifying glass and felt sad. She didn't like what she saw – her behavior was deceitful, manipulative, bad… It wasn't a sudden realization, but rather one that developed over time and grew ever stronger until the time when Korrie was forced to consider that perhaps she had made some mistakes. And perhaps she could *fix them*.

Willingly "backing herself into a corner," Korrie went to the principal's office and sat down. There was no place to run. Even if she fled the office, fled her school, fled her whole town, she could never flee from herself. She took a deep breath and told the principal that she was sorry for her behavior in school. She took responsibility for a lot of her poor choices. She then apologized to specific teachers whom she had hurt in her moments of rule-breaking and general disrespect. She braced herself for stern lectures and condemnation… but it never came. Her principal and teachers told her what a strong, beautiful woman she was and how much she had to offer. She worked hard during the remainder of the school year and really turned her act around. Korrie found that there are other ways to get what she wants other than to lie and go against the rules – and in fact those methods *didn't* ultimately work for her. She learned that people wouldn't hate her for admitting she was wrong. And she discovered that her reputation was hers alone and that by consistently maintaining positive changes, she *could* regain the trust of others.

She also found out that she herself had the potential to trust others. As she progressed in therapy, Korrie began to accept her feelings – all of her feelings – and she internalized that people would not slap her across the face for showing her emotions. It is okay to feel and express it. Korrie was angry about a lot of things. She felt abandoned and alone after significant people in her life had left. Her friends, it seemed, were all transient. Korrie never knew whom she could trust to care about her and stay around, so subconsciously she pushed everyone away in order to avoid the issue altogether. She told herself that things could be different, just as they were at school now. It may not happen today or tomorrow, but slowly, steadily, she would make it happen.

Perhaps the single greatest thing we can do for ourselves is to monitor our self-talk and keep it healthy and positive. Obviously this includes being nice to yourself and not telling yourself how "stupid" or "incompetent" you feel you are. Positive self-talk indeed *can* improve your self-image and boost your confidence. But this concept is much more far-reaching than that. It also impacts your effectiveness in handling various situations. For example, let's say that you're driving during rush hour and suddenly a car darts out from behind, loses control, and spins out dangerously close to your own vehicle. If you tell yourself, "Oh no! I'm doomed!" then you may have trouble thinking clearly as your panic escalates, leading to potentially increased danger. If, however, you remind yourself of what you learned in driving school – to lightly tap your breaks a few times before coming to a stop, then you can stop panic in its tracks, increasing the likelihood of a more positive outcome.

The things you tell yourself directly impact the way in which you view the world, not simply your attitudes and beliefs about yourself *within* the world, but also about the world and life in general. If you constantly engage in inner complaints about the state of your workplace, your family and friends, and life in general, then it follows that your worldview will be a negative one, regardless of your feelings about *yourself*.

In Korrie's story above, more needed changing than just her reputation. The only way she was able to take the necessary steps towards changing her reputation was to first modify her self-messages. Where she once told herself, "No one will ever accept me if I make a mistake," and "I can't trust anyone because they will leave me anyway," she now told herself, "People will respect me for admitting when I'm wrong," and "Perhaps I can relearn to trust others like others are relearning to trust me." These two changes drastically changed Korrie's worldview and helped her make better choices, ultimately leading to a more peaceful life. She saw there were problems and she saw which problems were hers to fix. She saw opportunity to improve her life and she grabbed the chance.

The beauty of self-talk is that through it you create yourself and consequently your world. If you tell yourself there are options, there will be. If you tell yourself there are good people out there, you will find them. If you view the world as bright and positive and full of opportunity, then for you it will be true. Your perception *is* your reality.

Chapter 4

CONFRONTING TRIGGERS

"A slip is not a relapse and a
relapse is not the end."

– *Common saying*

It was the dreaded moment that nearly everyone with an eating disorder history fears. The scenario so many of us try desperately to avoid. A new twist in the already winding labyrinth of recovery. It was about a month before my move to Florida to begin graduate school and I was at my last appointment with my medical doctor in Ohio. My doctor looked at her files as a number escaped her lips – a number indicating that my weight had gone above my ideal weight range.

I looked at my doctor and stated plainly, "That is a problem for me."

She asked me to verbally run through what I eat on a typical day. *Was this really happening? How did I let it come to this?* I wondered frantically to myself as I began listing foods. My doctor and I entered into a conversation about my meal plan and intuitive eating. On the outside I was nodding and agreeing with what my doctor told me. On the inside however, it was a bit more of a struggle.

A few minutes into the talk I realized that I wasn't hearing my doctor clearly. I recognized that the actual words she spoke were being distorted by my raging eating disorder thoughts. I silently vowed to lose weight. I would try to do it in a healthy way, but I couldn't stand to see the number on the scale so high. I left her office determined to succeed with my new self-imposed diet.

Then a funny thing happened – over the next several weeks my weight continued to climb! It was about a month after I moved to Florida that I put on a pair of jeans that used to fit me loosely and suddenly became aware that they were too tight. Cursing out all pants, I took them off and strengthened my resolve to lose weight. But as the evening wore on I found myself constantly drawn to the kitchen. I was bored so I ate. I was sad so I ate. In all honesty I *was* "hungry" – but not for food. I was hungry for balance, for friendship, for love, for a routine that felt manageable.

At my next therapy appointment I got honest about my struggles. Together we decided that I should go back to the basics for a while. Meal planning. Mechanical eating. Consciously listening to physical cues of hunger and satiety. My new therapist in Florida did not think I was out of control, which was my fear. He told me to relax and be kinder to myself. Transitions are hard. Being overly self-critical would only make it harder.

I took charge of my eating habits – I ate when I was hungry, I stopped when I was full. I made every attempt to get nutritional variety in my diet. Sometimes it was difficult, especially on days when I came home tired or had a lot of work to do, but I kept chugging along because recovery was important to me. I'll be honest – there were ups and downs and at one point, about a year after I moved to Florida, I had to address my weight with my doctor. Although I knew I was slowly approaching the highest end of my healthy weight range and although I *wanted* to settle back down to my natural set-point, I cried my eyes out at that appointment.

My doctor and I discussed my eating and exercise habits. Three years into recovery I was still not exercising much, even though at this point I was medically able – and even advised – to get my activity level up. Living alone and maintaining a busy schedule of work, school, writing, and volunteer work – not to mention my social activities – I had gradually settled into an unhealthy, even sedentary, lifestyle. I sat at my desk all day at work and in class, and then at my dining room table at home as I completed my work for the next day. There was very little physical activity involved.

And then there were my eating habits. I had long work-school-social-life days. I usually came home at night exhausted and ready to go to bed. Over time I had grown lazier about grocery shopping and cooking, preferring items from the frozen food section over healthier options that required more prep time. My nutritional variety suffered and I began to feel it. I was somewhat more tired and sluggish than I had once been and felt anxiety over my weight.

I will point out however that my weight concerns were not terribly disordered. They were motivated in large part by a healthy desire for physical fitness and the vigor and energy that accompany it. True, there was still that small voice in my head shouting that *this is the perfect opportunity for a complete makeover! I can lose weight and totally redesign my body!* You know… *that* voice.

As the discussion with my doctor continued I felt very sad. She told me hard truths that I did not want to hear. They were uncomfortable and annoying and they boiled down to the following statement: *I am in the same boat as all the "normal people" out there who have to eat right and exercise to remain in a healthy range.* Irritating, right? I know!

It was a difficult thing to hear after a seven-year battle against my eating disorder and three years in recovery. I was no longer "sick." I was no longer "special" in that I was exempt from exercise. My body was healthy and needed to be properly cared for in order to *stay* healthy. We developed a plan so that I would be able to fine-tune my eating and exercise habits. This would not be a "diet." There would be no going overboard. There would be balance and clear guidelines about my food intake and exercise. Not too much, not too little. Balance. And I would continue to meet with my treatment team to monitor my progress.

As you may suspect, the issue of balance – especially in relation to eating and exercise habits – was still a point of contention. I fought with all I had in the first few days to break away from all-or-nothing thinking. It was hard and I struggled. It was my toughest struggle against my eating disorder thoughts since my recovery began three-and-a-half years before. During that first week my thoughts, feelings, and behaviors slowly slipped into the realm of the eating disorder and from there positioned themselves into a downward spiral, rapidly crashing down, down, down! After only a few days, I felt happy, motivated, excited – "high." And in one moment, as I prepared for class, I recognized that it was all coming from an unhealthy place.

The height of clarity came on a Tuesday evening as I took my seat in a psychopathology class. That was when I knew that I had to do something fast to save and protect my recovery. Glancing up at my professor every so often and pretending to take notes, I wrote myself a letter. It was a letter from my healthy self to my slipping self, about the difference between having an eating disorder and living life. For the first time, I wasn't imagining anyone else's voice sharing these thoughts. I wasn't channeling my inner-therapist or nutritionist or parents or friends. The letter was truly from *me*, and the thoughts contained within were my strong beliefs. They rang true. And as such, when I reread the letter, I heard the message loud and clear:

Dear Naomi,

Since you're already slipping a bit into unhealthy thoughts and behaviors, I thought you might like to hear from that little healthy voice again. So hi, that's me. And I'm going to tell it like it is, so get ready:

You are skating on a melting pond. This might sound fun and exciting to you now – losing weight, seeing that number on the scale drop, feeling that "high" from not eating enough. But remember this: It always *sounds fun and exciting. At* first. *But follow it through to the end and you'll wind up with nothing. No happiness, no peace, no master's degree, no money, no dream job, no positive relationships. No marriage, no children, no hobbies, the list goes on and on. And get this – no weight loss either! Whatever you lose will just come back (when you eventually recover again) and probably more.*

And don't think that the answer is going back into treatment again. Maybe it seems like a comforting thought to you, but even if it's everything and more that your experience at Renfrew was in 2007, follow that *through to the end... After treatment you go home – what, did you think you'd get to stay forever? And, you won't get to go home to your apartment or your job or your school or even to others' trust. You'll go home to a shattered life which you will have to fight – uphill all the way – to rebuild. Your life as you know it will be gone. You'll have nothing.*

Think about what you want. Think about your dreams. You want to work at Company X. You've wanted it for years. It's finally possible, but if you mess it up you will not get another chance! *What is more important to you? Your desire to work at Company X is a dream, a passion. Your desire to lose weight is an illness, an obsession. Even if this comes down to something that simple – the choice between the job you want and chasing that ever-lower number on the scale – consider your options. Think. While you still can.*

At your lowest weight you wrote yourself a letter about the misery of anorexia. It was torture. There was nothing in your life that you enjoyed, nothing you looked forward to. Don't go there again. Discuss this in therapy. Work hard. You always tell people that they don't need to relapse in order to do the work. It's true for you as well. You're good *at residential work. You've mastered the art of pulling out of a terrible relapse. But doing it again won't make you stronger. You'll just be playing a rerun. Nothing real. And eventually it'll get old and boring and you'll burn out, too exhausted to fight. And then you're lost and it will take a miracle to bring you back. In short, life will utterly suck.*

But here's the good news: You're still okay. You're still healthy and you still have tremendous opportunity in front of you. The world is your oyster. You can have anything, go anywhere, be anything of your choosing. But if you choose diets and weight-loss you are inviting anorexia back into your life and essentially handing it your life on a silver platter. Don't be stupid.

You do need to get back on track with your food and exercise, but you have to be really, really careful. And you cannot *do it alone. Trust your therapist. She knows these things better than you do. Ask her to guide you. Be honest with your parents. Use your support system. Reach out and ask for help. You* can't *do this alone. You do* not *know what you're doing. It will* never *be "just a diet." Give it up. I know it's hard, I know it's frustrating and disappointing. This is one of those times you need to sit with your feelings, self-soothe, and* accept. *Don't chase what you're missing, cherish what you have.*

Love, Naomi

I took this letter to my next therapy appointment and reread it often as I struggled to pull out of the downward spiral and achieve true balance for possibly the first time in my life. In the beginning, when I was trying to overcome anorexic eating patterns, I needed to be told that there was no upper limit to what I could eat. That was what I needed for survival. I needed permission to eat, permission to meet my own needs, and permission to enjoy my world. But that was black-and-white too, and even though it helped me get to a much healthier place, it was not the answer in and of itself.

As I recovered I found myself having a field day with food. I could eat this! And this! And this! Eating disorders are traumatic. In recovery, it was as if I had to continually prove to myself that I wouldn't starve again. If there was food, I found myself eating it even when I didn't really want it. I just had to have a "little bit" because then I wouldn't feel deprived. I was terrified of deprivation. Having lived for years in a self-imposed prison with strict rules and denial of even my most basic needs, I desperately craved the comfort and reassurance that it was over now and that I was safe, and nurtured, and that my needs were met.

After I wrote myself the recovery letter, I wrote another one to give voice to the eating disorder thoughts. I decided to "hear them out" and see if there was any truth within them. (In parentheses are the rational thoughts that I knew contained the truth even as I wrote this letter.)

Dear Naomi,

I want to lose weight and now I finally can! It's even doctor-approved and everything! I "have" to lose weight, diet, and exercise. (Is that really *what the doctor said?) How exciting! My body is my project, it's my own art project that I get to decide what it looks like and how big it is. (As if that is going to work!) And I* know *that when I'm smaller, I will be happier, more peaceful, more energized! (Who here hasn't heard that before from "Ed"?) I'm already energized! (Read: "Manic") Look at me, I barely need to sleep, I'm high-powered, I feel great. So motivated! So free! (So MANIC!) The familiar "rules" are coming back to me. ("Ed" nearly has me in his clutches again.) I know how to lose the weight, I know how to be healthier. (By re- reading my other letter.) I can do this, trust me, I know what I'm doing! (Yes, I know this path all too well…) It's amazing, almost surreal! (Maybe that's because it's not real.) I'm so in charge! (The illusion of control takes over when I know deep down that I'm losing control.)*

The letter stopped there. I couldn't continue because there was nothing more to say. The eating disorder was empty. It was devoid of any real passion or insight. It just wanted what it wanted and it wanted it now. Chasing an impossible, ever-elusive goal – that's all it was. As happy as I am that I wrote the recovery letter, I am equally happy I wrote the eating disorder letter. It showed me in a very real way that the urges and compulsions to act out on eating disorder symptoms were coming from an unhealthy place of extremes. I began taking little steps to find balance. Not just in food and exercise, but in all areas.

The first example was that when I drove in my car and the temperature was too hot or too cold, I began changing the air up or down by one or two notches at a time, rather than all the way to hot or all the way to cold. I used to think that if I changed the temperature drastically that I would feel more comfortable more quickly. What actually happened was that I went from "too hot" to "too cold" and back again, usually for the duration of my drive.

It might sound like a silly example, but I think it is symbolic of the way I was living my life. Jumping from one extreme to the other never satisfied me and it never evened itself out. It was true of the time I spent on schoolwork, my diet and exercise habits, and the temperature in my car. So the next time I met with my therapist, we began working towards the goal of balance. First and foremost we addressed my diet and exercise habits and established a healthy routine.

The goal – above and beyond the literal improvements in diet and exercise – was for me to take a more active role in promoting balance in my own life. Just because I had to modify my eating and exercise habits didn't mean I had to go overboard on either. Of course not, that's silly! I made better choices at the grocery store than I had made previously, and I began to slowly incorporate exercise into my week. My routine shifted to incorporate increased cooking time so that I could prepare home cooked meals for myself. I took the time to take care of my body through exercise. I used to think I was always "too busy" for these things. But if there's one thing I know about time management, it's that you make time for the things that matter to you. I had to get my priorities in check.

Gradually, my team told me, my weight would settle back down and my body would return to its natural set-point. During this period of "basics" I would not attempt to control my weight and I would not "aim" for any specific numbers. I would continue to only weigh myself in my therapist's office and each time we would discuss what the number signified to me.

Korrie

"Tolerance is the key to dealing with triggers," says Korrie. "You can't avoid them – you can just learn to deal with them."

Korrie works at a high-end clothing store. Frequently, insensitive customers ask her what size clothing she wears. Korrie used to feel immensely triggered by this, and often still does, especially when the customer responds even more inappropriately. One incident in particular stands out in Korrie's mind.

A woman walked into the store and looked her up and down.

"What size do you wear?" she asked Korrie.

"Excuse me?" Korrie replied.

"What. Size. Do. You. Wear?" the woman obnoxiously "clarified." Backed into a corner and unable to dodge such a direct question (at her supervisor's direction), Korrie reluctantly answered the customer. It turned out that the woman wanted to know Korrie's size because "I have a granddaughter about your size and I want to buy her a gift!" But when the woman heard Korrie's clothing size, she gaped in disbelief and said, "Oh, *really?*"

Korrie went home that evening wanting to engage in symptoms. She forced herself to refrain and to use distraction skills instead. She also used a DBT skill and "took a nonjudgmental approach."

"It used to bother me a lot more than it does now when these things would happen," says Korrie. "But now I realize that they are just customers who don't think before they speak. It's still annoying. But just because they perceive something doesn't mean they know. They *don't* know! What they choose to do with the information I tell them is their business. It's their boundary issues, not mine."

Korrie's clothing size was none of her customers' business, but nonetheless they crossed a boundary by asking, again and again. Although these grown women (and men) should know better, they acted insensitively and caused pain without intending to, or even realizing!

Numbers are a common trigger. Eating disorders are replete with numbers. Weight, calories, blood pressure, pulse. My therapist once asked me to spend some time thinking about what the numbers mean to me. It was a difficult assignment because in focusing so hard for so long on the numbers, I had neglected to ever consider *why* they were so important! I shared the assignment with my mother, who could see my situation more objectively than I could, and she responded immediately, "Maybe the numbers are so important to you because they are an absolute measuring stick."

What an idea!

My eating disorder distorted my body image, my sense of self, and my ideas of perfection. My ability to measure these things was terribly skewed. One minute I thought I looked fine, the next horrible. The numbers gave me a sense of stability. In thinking about why numbers are so triggering to so many people I realized that grasping onto numbers is a way to grasp onto constancy – to attempt to hold onto something stable when everything else seems so chaotic.

It is precisely in moments of chaos – real or perceived – that people in recovery from eating disorders struggle the most. According to Rebekah Bardwell Doweyko transitions are the most severe triggers. In my case this meant moving away from my family and the place I'd lived most of my life to a new town where I would make new friends, have a new job, go to a new school, and have to develop a new routine. Because everything was suddenly so new, it made sense that I longed for things that were familiar. Sometimes when people experience major transitions, especially those that challenge their existing notions of how life should be, they do experience immense struggles, and sometimes slip or even relapse. A slip is not a relapse and a relapse is not the end. Pick yourself up, get the help you need, and keep moving forward.

✐ Taylor

Taylor was working as a contractor when she needed an invasive medical procedure. After her surgery and during her recovery period she worried about her future at the company. After all, her main goal in recovery from her eating disorder was to be able to build up a new life – to be able to have a life and a job. Her recruiter assured her that she was fine, but a week later Taylor received a phone call from her employer saying that the company was not renewing her contract.

Feeling like a massive failure, Taylor felt that the one thing she'd worked so hard for in recovery was taken from her. Her job was gone. Her medical insurance was gone. Her new identity, it seemed, was gone.

"My self-esteem went into a fragile state," Taylor recounts, "I felt like I had nothing left to stay healthy for and I deteriorated at an alarming rate, faster and faster until eventually I had to go into residential treatment."

After her inpatient stay, Taylor returned to the workforce, this time to a different job with a different boss with an even lower tolerance for employee struggles. After a difficult night during which Taylor had to call the police on a dangerous former roommate, Taylor came to work exhausted. During her lunch break, she fell asleep in her car and was caught by her supervisor. She was called into the office and questioned. Taylor, at her wit's end, broke down sobbing. She dealt with it, finished off the day and went home.

The following day the manager told her that she wouldn't be penalized for attendance reasons, but she would receive a misconduct warning which essentially meant that she couldn't receive a promotion for a full calendar year. This time, rather than blame herself too harshly, Taylor recognized that, yes, she made a mistake, but the consequences imposed by her manager were only applicable if she stayed with the company.

She refused to beat herself up over it, and instead decided to take immediate action. Taylor updated her resume, went on interviews, and landed an even better job at which she was much happier. This time, the transition was much smoother.

Before my move to Florida I did not truly understand that all eating disorder symptoms are so similar. I knew to be on the lookout for my old eating disorder patterns – restricting and over-exercising – but I did not realize that I would be susceptible to picking up other symptoms, such as emotional overeating. Because I was working honestly with my therapist I was able to nip this "new" problem in the bud and focus on making sense of my new life – organizing my apartment, setting up a bank account, setting up a school and work routine… the things that *really* needed to be addressed and were temporarily covered up by my food concerns. In time I adapted to my new routine, I made friends, I learned to keep house on my own, and I succeeded at my new school and job.

My approach to dealing with triggers has become increasingly more functional with time. I know what I need to do *and* I have enough practice actually *doing it* that I can usually take a step back and see the situation honestly and shamelessly, using my skills to help me through. But just what do you do when you're struggling with your motivation to overcome triggers? What do you do when it seems that the number on the scale measures your achievement, your character, your worth?

Breaking through triggers and strengthening motivation can often be jump-started by creative exercises in which you symbolically free yourself from negativity. One such project that has recently gained in popularity is the "scale smash." It's exactly as it sounds – you take a scale, preferably the one taunting you, and you smash it along with all the misery it contains.

Lexi

Over the years during which Lexi struggled with her eating disorder, her scale had become her life while simultaneously sucking the life out of her. One day in group therapy someone brought up the scale smash but it was not feasible for Lexi at that point. Lexi's scale had been confiscated by her best friend some time earlier because she saw that Lexi was using it in a self-destructive way.

Every summer when she was in college, Lexi met up with her sorority sisters for a weekend of fun and relaxation on the lake where they would catch up on the details of each others' lives. Lexi looked forward to it every year, but there was also a sense of anxiety during the summer after her junior year. By this time Lexi had been in treatment for a couple of months and had undergone changes both physically and emotionally. Even though her sorority sisters knew about her treatment, she was still greatly concerned about how they would react to seeing her. What would they say? Would they expect her to be perfectly cured? Would they be disappointed in her for not being completely symptom-free? And in addition to their reactions, how would Lexi herself manage spending time wearing a bathing suit at the lake? Her only comfort on the long drive to the weekend gathering was that she would see her best friend, the girl who took her scale and who had encouraged her to begin therapy in the first place.

The first afternoon she was in town for the weekend, Lexi met up with her best friend for dinner. During the meal Lexi shared what she had learned about the scale smash and asked her friend where the scale had been "hiding" for several months now. At first her friend laughed at her, thinking it was just another ploy on Lexi's part to take back her scale. But after some discussion her friend not only agreed to let her smash the scale, but she also wanted to help!

Lexi sat with the scale for a few moments, permanent markers in hand. It was difficult to "deface" the scale with the first word, but once she started writing she knew exactly what she wanted to say. She wanted the truth!

"I am strong!"

"Ultimately I will win!"

"You do not control me!"

"I will fight!"

"Just a number, that's all you are!"

Lexi wrote and wrote. She wrote on the place where she used to stand to weigh herself. She wrote on the sides. She wrote on the plastic cover over the numbers. Then she took the scale outside with a hammer. Lexi and her best friend took turns bashing in the scale, smashing it as hard as they could. At first a few dents were made, but then pieces started flying off. The plastic covering the numbers flew about ten feet! The top separated from the bottom! Springs detached!

Lexi left her friend's house that night feeling she had put an important piece of her past behind her. The scale had been her greatest comfort and her greatest restraint. It was her best friend and worst enemy. Now the scale was just a pile of mangled metal and broken plastic. Lexi was free. Now it was time to go have fun with her sorority sisters!

Chapter 5

TREATING FOOD AS MEDICINE

"The type of food you reach for is a
window into your emotional world."

— Jodi Krumholz

By now it should be sufficiently clear that, at their core, eating disorders are not about food consumption, or lack thereof. However, in a disorder where food is medicine it would be not only unreasonable but also irresponsible to ignore food as a major factor of recovery. Issues pertaining to healthy eating and healthy attitudes and relationships with food cannot and should not be overlooked. When people first enter a state of recovery, it is very common for them to feel as though they are standing on shaky ground – or, more accurately, as Dr. Jen Nardozzi often puts it, that they are standing on shaky *legs*. Just as a baby giraffe wobbles and stumbles as it learns to walk in the moments after birth, an individual newly in recovery must be prepared for the unsteady first moments of health. This challenging beginning is a critical turning point requiring a great deal of perseverance and resilience.

Most likely there will be slips – and it is appropriate to learn from them and increase your efforts to avoid such setbacks in the future – but at no point is it acceptable to get down on yourself and give up hope. It is so important to stay positive and work your recovery step by step. Each success builds a foundation for another and another. Going into the beginning stages of recovery, it is important to have a realistic understanding of the process of recovery, especially in regards to the specific actions needed to maintain your health.

Working with a nutritionist who specializes in eating disorders is absolutely key. Many men and women recovering from eating disorders hesitate to seek the help of a nutritionist, despite the overwhelming importance of nutrition in achieving a solid state of recovery. Even after working with a nutritionist as part of a treatment team – perhaps in an inpatient or residential setting – people are less likely to follow through on seeing a nutritionist long term than they are to follow through on seeing a therapist. Upon reaching the early stages of recovery, a person's nutritionist tends to be the first one "kicked off the team."

Jodi Krumholz, director of nutrition for the Renfrew Center, claims that one explanation for this phenomenon is that it is possible for you to be *too knowledgeable* about nutrition! This is dangerous for a couple of reasons. First, if you know a tremendous amount of information about nutrition, then you may be less inclined to listen to a nutritionist because you feel you "know better than they do." This kind of thinking can potentially lead to power struggles. Second, you may consider it a waste of time and money to go to appointments where you doubt you will come away with anything new.

"Many people feel on some level that they aren't going to get more knowledge of nutrition from a nutritionist," says Jodi Krumholz. While this may be true – *in part* – it is inconsequential in terms of keeping up with nutrition appointments. "The biggest role of nutritionists is to hold the patient accountable and support the patient in recovery," Jodi continues. Regardless of whether or not the nitty-gritty details of nutrition must be learned (such as why the body needs from each nutrient), the aspects of support and accountability are essential.

"For a long period of time, the patient needs someone to do this for them," says Jodi, "It takes a long time before somebody can fly on their own."

Your nutritionist will be able to develop a meal plan to meet your specific dietary needs and may help you learn to monitor your own eating through the use of food journals. A food journal is a form you fill out after each meal and snack. It will generally have a section to write down what foods you ate, the nutritional content (usually in exchanges, where a certain number of grams of a nutrient equals one exchange of that nutrient). Food journals also typically have a rating scale for hunger-satiety and a space to journal about your thoughts and feelings about the meal. Your nutritionist may initially ask you to record every meal and review your food journals in session. In time, you may taper to recording one meal per day or recording a few days per week, until such time that you no longer need the food journals.

While there are many different issues that people identify through keeping food journals, eventually certain patterns tend to emerge. A few common issues include emotional overeating and emotional under-eating, mindful eating and mindless eating, and routine eating and special-occasion eating. All three of these areas are interwoven such that tackling one is a stepping stone towards tackling the next.

Taylor

Taylor binged for the first time at the age of ten. She recalls only having one or two experiences of eating as much as she possibly could, but many instances in which she would overindulge on food.

"For me, overeating isn't maniacal," says Taylor, "I would just eat… and then keep eating." It usually started small, with a small piece of cake or chocolate or other dessert item. Trouble arose because this small dessert was surrounded by hoards of other desserts. For example, if there was a large chocolate cake and Taylor took one small piece, it was difficult for her to be satisfied with her small piece when she knew that the rest of the cake was temptingly nearby.

After eating her piece of cake, Taylor would casually walk by the rest of the cake. She'd glance around to be sure that no one was looking. If no one noticed, then Taylor would stealthily help herself to another piece of cake. And after that, another and another.

"I was always ashamed afterwards. It usually happened over the course of twenty minutes, when I'd have that one piece of cake but then still be thinking about the cake. Sugary foods were my downfall. Dessert was something I always wanted and I felt like no matter how much I ate I would never have enough of it, I would never be satisfied, I would never know when I'd consumed 'enough.'"

The excuses were readily available:

"I won't eat later so it's okay."

"This will give me a nice burst of energy."

"It's reduced-fat or nonfat so it doesn't matter how much I eat."

"It's just this once, so it doesn't really count."

As with any behavior requiring a mountain of excuses, Taylor's food-related activities were a source of great shame. A lot of people with similar struggles experience eating as a way to "stuff down their feelings." For Taylor, binging and overeating served the same purpose as restricting and under-eating. It was a place for her to put her feelings, a distraction, and a way to numb the pain. The food was how Taylor subconsciously attempted to fill a need, even when she wasn't hungry. It wasn't a nutritional need. It was an emotional need.

Even when she restricted all other foods, Taylor still could not get enough dessert. No matter how full she was, she always needed more. She felt like if she started eating dessert, then she would never stop. After overindulging, Taylor would feel guilty and ashamed and desperate to "undo" her overeating through other symptoms, which in turn only caused her to think about food *more*. It was a vicious cycle.

"I never really figured out what, if anything, my overeating was trying to accomplish. I never really figured out *why* I did it. I just really, really liked dessert."

Taylor still doesn't know exactly what her overeating was about, but she does know that regardless of the reasons behind it, she still got better. Through the use of mechanical eating and changing her eating disorder "rules," Taylor created a new mindset for herself. A mindset in which dessert wasn't forbidden, but rather okay and good in moderation.

Emotional over or under-eating is often at the center of food-related difficulties. Whether or not one has a diagnosable eating disorder, the tangling of emotions and food is in itself a problem. What a lot of people do not understand is that emotional overeating and under-eating to avoid emotions are essentially two sides of the same coin. They may result in different health problems, weights, and stigmas, but at their core they are the same: Food is used as a form of self-medication. This Band-Aid fix only serves to cover up problems but does absolutely nothing to solve them. In actuality, using food this way only causes greater, more dangerous crises and exacerbates the original problem by weakening your ability to properly cope. As a result you will be more likely to turn to food to ease your distress, and in turn, less able to pull out of the cycle.

Let's say you're stuck in this pattern and want to get out. Maybe you can no longer determine your levels of hunger and fullness. Or maybe you do not feel satisfied, even after consuming a large amount of food. Jodi Krumholz advises that the best thing to do in these instances is to eat mechanically, which will be discussed later. Jodi also suggests journaling as a means of appropriate exploration. This can be done through the use of food journals.

In regards to a situation in which a person doesn't feel satisfied even when they have sufficiently eaten, and is perhaps even physically full to the point of discomfort, Jodi explains that food journals can help you understand what else is going on – emotionally. Food journals are an especially helpful form of journaling in this instance because through them you can begin to make connections between your feelings and types of foods. For example, do you tend to eat macaroni and cheese or sweet potatoes when you feel lonely? Do you chew gum or eat a lot of candy when you're anxious?

"The type of food you reach for is a window into your emotional world," says Jodi Krumholz. "Notice where your hunger is coming from," she clarifies. If your hunger is coming from your mouth, it might be an indication of anxiety. Eating chewy and sweet foods can have a calming effect and are thus used to "treat" the anxiety. If the hunger originates from your chest, that tends to signify a need for nurturance. By taking a moment to step back and notice where your hunger is coming from – that is, what emotions you are experiencing – sometimes sitting with uncomfortable feelings of anxiety and loneliness, you will be better able to meet your needs in a real way.

Obviously true physical hunger for food does not come from either your mouth or your chest, so if you feel the hunger coming from these places, that is a clear sign that it is an *emotional hunger.* A more detailed discussion on this topic can be found in the book *Nourishing Wisdom,* by Marc David. A qualified nutritionist will be able to help you address these issues in a healthy way.

There are many reasons why people overeat or under-eat. Jodi explains that these behaviors are typically present in individuals who seek to "numb out" and avoid feeling their emotions.

"On the surface," she says, "there is a lot of pressure to be thin in our society, but really it's about people not being able to cope with feelings." She goes on to explain that life is difficult – for anybody – and some people turn to food in order to cope. Binging and overeating, as in bulimia or binge eating disorder, are ways to numb out by "stuffing feelings down." Under-eating, as in anorexia, is a way to "restrict feelings."

Jodi cautions that an awareness of the underlying reasons behind your eating disorder symptoms is important to explore, as they can have detrimental effects in other areas of your life as well. If you recover from bulimia and then turn to alcohol or drugs, or gambling, or shopping sprees, or to *any* excessive indulgence, then you run the risk of "trading addictions." When this happens, you essentially give up your current external symptoms but replace them with new ones that are equally – or more – harmful and unhealthy. Overindulgence as a way to numb your feelings is a common theme that many men and women battling bulimia struggle against.

Conversely, those battling anorexia struggle on the opposite side of the spectrum. Restricting food becomes a way to escape feelings, but it goes much deeper than that. Whereas people struggling with bulimia tend to numb out by overdoing it, those dealing with anorexia tend to numb out through restriction – of food, of feelings, of life.

"When you restrict food you restrict life," says Jodi. "You don't go out with friends, you don't enjoy holidays. You can't get pleasure from meals with friends and family. You miss out on every special opportunity that involves food." There is such an extreme fear of having needs and of overindulging. There are also many cognitive distortions in place, such as black-and-white thinking. So as a result, these men and women go to the nth-degree to avoid meeting even their basic needs. I once came across a heartbreaking statement summing up this aspect of this particular eating disorder: "If I eat anything, I will eat everything... so I eat nothing." If this quote hits close to home, it is indicative of a serious problem. Please seek help.

It's important to make mention of the fact that not *all* emotional eating is unhealthy. As with virtually everything in life, moderation is the key. One example, says Jodi, is eating certain foods that remind you of a lost loved one when you miss them. This kind of emotional eating, *in moderation*, can help you feel connected to your loved one. Obviously if you have – or have had – an eating disorder, this is probably not a method of connection you would do well to consider. There are other ways, like listening to familiar songs or purchasing a perfume or cologne that reminds you of the person or, perhaps most fulfilling, emulating their positive qualities and carrying on their legacy (for more on grief, see Chapter 9).

One way that this kind of emotional eating can easily get out of hand is if you find yourself using food as a way to escape back to an earlier point in time when life was more pleasant and peaceful. This will most likely lead you down a dangerous path of numbing behaviors, eventually resulting in the return of obsessive thoughts regarding food, calories, weight, and other numbers.

If you are struggling with an active eating disorder or you are in the early stages of recovery, you may wonder how it is even possible not to think about food and body image and numbers all of the time. While breaking away from this mindset takes effort – and a lot of time – you can and will make it happen with practice and determination. Don't be discouraged if there are slips and setbacks. Use each struggle as an opportunity to dig deeper. Work *with*, not against, your nutritionist.

Jessica

One morning in residential treatment Jessica woke up happy. She looked in the mirror and loved what she saw. She still felt heavy and was uncomfortable with that, but she saw true happiness and went into the day with the greatest attitude. Then she met with her nutritionist.

"Jessica," her nutritionist started, "I'm concerned about your weight. It's gone up a bit over the last few days. Let's take a moment to discuss what could be going on."

Jessica felt her heart sink.

Her nutritionist continued flipping through her charts and found that Jessica had recently been prescribed a new medication which sometimes causes weight gain as a side effect. Her nutritionist seemed more at ease, but Jessica flew into a panic. Her thoughts raced – cut out calories. Exercise. Anything it takes to lose the weight!

"How could you let this happen?!" she shouted at her nutritionist as a raging torrent of anger and hurt welled up inside of her. Jessica left the session discouraged and ready to leave treatment early. She immediately went to her room and changed into the largest items of clothing she had with her. Then she went on a rampage trying to find her best friend at the treatment center, a girl named Aimee.

Well Aimee seems to have disappeared off the face of the earth Jessica thought in frustrated annoyance. At one point Aimee walked right past Jessica, but Jessica didn't see her because of the tears pouring from her eyes and because of her sudden preoccupation with her weight and body image. She eventually found Aimee and together they went to art therapy (see Chapter 7), after which Jessica sat down to write a (quite uncensored) letter to her nutritionist. It began, "What the fuck were you thinking?!" and went on for three solid pages in which Jessica rambled on and on about how she hated her nutritionist and how she would never trust her again. She wrote that she'd been working on allowing herself to choose additional snacks and desserts but that now she would never go beyond the bare minimum that was required of her.

Jessica hated that she let her weight completely ruin her day. She realized that her eating disorder still had her in its clutches even though she'd been happy the day before. She was determined to work through this and the next day Jessica had a breakthrough.

Rather than wake up in a good mood, Jessica woke up in a *balanced* mood. As she considered the events of the day before more calmly and objectively than she had previously, she realized that she was the same person before she walked into her nutritionist's office as she was after. Although she had cried for three hours straight after her appointment, she was the same Jessica that had put a smile on the face of everyone she came in contact with prior to her nutrition meeting.

Says Jessica, "How could a number change so much so fast? It didn't make sense. When I reflected on the day before, I saw that my weight didn't define me as a person. It couldn't – I was the same person as I was at a different weight, but the number was different, so obviously it couldn't define me."

That morning Jessica went back to her room to change her clothing once again, only this time she changed back into her regular clothes. She admits to being astonished that they still fit, despite the fact that she'd worn them yesterday, but she set those thoughts aside and focused instead on the thought that a number cannot magically make her a happier person. She still looked the same, felt the same, and laughed the same. Nothing had really changed about her except for the number on the scale.

In working with her nutritionist she further developed her breakthrough.

"I'd been defined by numbers my entire life," Jessica explains, "Grades, batting averages, fielding percentages, etc. etc. etc." Upon exploring what these numbers meant in her life, Jessica was finally able to move forward towards a day when numbers would no longer define her.

Jessica maintains that with her nutritionist's help she "overcame the stronghold numbers had on her all because of a little mix-up and miscommunication about a medication."

After this incident, Jessica's nutritionist encouraged her to go back to choosing snacks and desserts she enjoyed. She responded to Jessica's angry letter with warmth and understanding, praising Jessica for coming a long way in learning to communicate her feelings. They worked through a rather painful episode together, using it as a springboard for growth. Jessica proceeded with the courage inherent in her personality, and continued along her path to recovery.

Mindful eating, or intuitive eating, is the ultimate food-related goal in recovering from any eating disorder. "Mindful eating" is a term that encompasses eating when hungry and stopping when full; a conscious awareness of taste and texture, quantity and quality; and an ability to trust one's own body.

Jodi Krumholz cautions that it takes a long time to get to a place where mindful eating is a reality. This is true even for people who have never struggled with an eating disorder in their lives. Jodi explains that this is due in part to cultural associations between food and certain activities. For example, many people eat large quantities of popcorn at movies. They may not even be hungry, but they associate movies with eating popcorn. The popcorn itself has become part and parcel of the movie-going *experience*. Often, especially when eating popcorn at a movie or eating dinner in front of the television, people will look down and realize they have just consumed a far greater amount of food than they had originally intended. They may not even remember eating that much at all.

"I think that the whole mindfulness concept really escapes most people," says Jodi. "So to really get back there, especially after you have had an eating disorder, can take years. For a long time to come I think that people are working with eating mechanically." Mechanical eating is the process of consciously and deliberately mimicking the behavior associated with mindful eating in a carefully controlled way.

Meals are planned out in accordance with a meal plan predetermined by a dietitian and food is consumed systematically – perhaps faster or slower than one's eating disorder would dictate, and with increased conscious awareness with regard to desisting from food rituals such as cutting foods into tiny pieces or mixing them inappropriately. Such behavior is common among those struggling with eating disorders and can really hinder recovery. Holding onto food rituals is a subconscious way for some people to hold onto the feelings of control that an eating disorder provides. Even when someone very badly wants recovery, it can be exceedingly difficult for them to relinquish control and to trust their treatment team. Holding onto food rituals, however, *will keep you stuck*. Giving up an eating disorder needs to be a complete giving up. That does not mean to say that it can't happen in stages, because it certainly can and there are many short-term goals and successes to be had along the way, but the eventual goal of recovery is to cease using eating disorder symptoms at *all*. In recovery, food is just food and feelings are just feelings.

Mechanical eating is very helpful in this regard because not only is it a way to manage behaviors, but it is also a helpful tool in overcoming distorted thoughts and easing uncomfortable feelings. Instead of worrying about how much is too much and what it means about you or your feelings to eat certain foods (e.g. that eating cake means you have no self-control) you can choose foods that you enjoy with the comfort of knowing that they fall within your meal plan.

A young woman named Melissa once shared with me how a fellow patient had helped her in treatment: Melissa had been choosing "safe" snacks and refusing any options that she viewed as "bad" or "junk" foods. Finally another woman in her treatment program told her that the nutritional value of each option was the same as the next. Snack option A was essentially the same as snack option B because the body will digest them and make use of the same nutrients from both. Viewing foods as an assortment of nutrients eliminated the self-judgments Melissa made about her eating and helped her allow herself to choose the snacks she truly wanted.

According to Jodi Krumholz, the intuitiveness required for successful mindful eating is twofold. The first part, as Melissa's story demonstrates, is knowing what food you really want, and being honest with yourself about it. The second aspect is to trust yourself to eat these foods in moderation.

Ask yourself, "Am I really hungry or do I just want to eat for XYZ reason?" Once you are able to differentiate between your reasons for eating (or not eating), and when you are able to determine your levels of hunger and fullness, then it is time to move towards trusting yourself. Just as trust in any relationship must be earned – especially in cases where the trust has eroded for whatever reason and must be re-earned – learning to trust yourself is a delicate process. Beyond matters of hunger and fullness, reasons for eating, and menu selections, lie issues of emotional trust. Are you still afraid of food? Are you afraid of weight gain? Are you afraid of weight loss? Are food and weight still your "shields" protecting you from a dangerous world? If so, then *you cannot be truly honest with yourself* and you should continue to eat mechanically. There is no shame in mechanical eating and it does not *at all* indicate weakness or sickness. On the contrary, it is an exceptionally wise and responsible choice. Most people in the world cannot truly eat intuitively, eating disorder or not! Some times will be easier than others; some meals will be easier than others. If you begin eating intuitively and then find that you are struggling, you would do well to return to the basics – at least temporarily – in order to regain your footing.

Korrie

When struggling through a meal, Korrie finds it helpful to take a step outside herself. She sets aside thoughts of meal plans and food journals and tries to adopt an outsider's perspective.

"What helps me is seeing it from someone else's view," she says. "I don't play distraction games so much or anything like that, but I think to myself that people eat all the time. They eat moderately and they survive. I'm no different. I can do the same."

On occasions when Korrie overeats, a little or a lot, she tends to feel guilty and ashamed and frustrated and desperate to "undo" it.

Korrie says, "When that happens, instead of purging I remind myself that people eat like this on holidays and birthdays and they wake up the next morning and still do what they need to do. They still are functioning. Life goes on."

Sometimes life goes on one meal at a time.

When you find yourself struggling through a meal, it is generally a good idea to use skills involving distraction. Whereas in a therapy session it is appropriate to confront your stress and work through it, meals are not the time and place for such work. When I was in the beginning stages of my recovery, I mistook healthy, *temporary*, distraction for avoidance, which is most certainly not the case. It may be helpful to consider the following scenario:

A soldier is on the battlefield and is shot in the leg. He can still walk but there is no denying that he needs medical care. Without treatment he runs the risk of serious infection, gangrene, and even death. Nonetheless, he is on the battlefield and there is no medical care readily available. What's more, if he stops to nurse his wounds he runs the even greater risk of being killed or captured by the enemy. Although his injury needs attention, now is not the time or the place for it. In fact, shifting his attention to his leg at this moment will almost certainly have detrimental effects. By choosing to focus on the battle at hand, rather than his wounds, the soldier is not practicing avoidance, but rather prioritization. He will seek medical care later, when it is safe.

In the beginning of your recovery you are like that soldier. Things are not perfect. No matter how much work you have done in therapy there will always be more issues, more layers beneath the surface, more discoveries to be made, and more work to be done. You may still be hurting inside. You may crave resolution to your problems immediately. Although all of this may be true, *mealtime is not the time*! Remember, you are like the soldier who must first achieve safety and *only then* seek medical attention. Resolving your issues *is* important, but in focusing on them at the wrong time you run the even greater risk of forfeiting your recovery. That may seem like an extreme statement, but you are probably familiar with the idea that acting on your symptoms one time makes it that much easier to slip again and again.

It's the same idea here – trying to work out all of your problems before eating can aid the mindset that, "I can only eat when I'm feeling okay." In this way you are in danger of rationalizing your way out of eating. There is a psychological term called "negative reinforcement." Contrary to popular belief, this does not mean punishment. What negative reinforcement actually means is that something unpleasant is taken away, and the absence of pain reinforces the behavior that led to its absence. If a meal causes you stress, and by leaving the table without eating your stress goes away, that will by definition reinforce your decision not to eat, making it more likely that you will do the same thing next time.

Recovery is like a muscle. Although at first it may be very challenging to use healthy coping skills – such as appropriate distraction – the more you practice using them, the stronger your recovery muscle grows. In time, recovery can become a very natural process. It can be hard to believe that at first, but I can tell you from experience that it does get easier. As illustrated in the anecdote in Chapter 6 about my friend's father's comment – without my sharing about my past, people do not even suspect that I had an eating disorder. Furthermore, despite the fact that there are still occasional struggles, there are also times that *I* am not even conscious that I had an eating disorder. It is a part of what shaped who I am today, but it is not the person I am today. Reaching this stage admittedly takes time and a whole lot of practice, practice, practice.

Getting back to the original discussion, what are some ways you can practice distraction skills when appropriate? There are a number of games that can be played at mealtime to help take your mind off of your stress so that it is easier to eat. Notice that these games can also alleviate stress, in a positive way. Most of these games can be divided into two categories – alphabet games and memory games.

An example of an alphabet game is a game in which one person names a category or theme, such as "picnic," and then each player takes a turn naming a different item starting with the proceeding letter of the alphabet. For example, in the category "picnic," items might include: **a**pple, **b**lanket, **c**hildren… and so on.

Another game using the alphabet involves choosing a theme, such as "Disney actors/actresses," and going around the table taking turns choosing a different name beginning with the last letter of the previous name. For example: Miley Cyru**s**, **S**elena Gome**z**, **Z**ac Efro**n**… and so on.

An entirely different alphabet game is one in which someone at the table begins by saying, "A." Then another person says, "B." A third says, "C." And so on until "Z." The challenge is that if two people speak at the same time, the group starts over from "A." Also, no one may say two letters in a row.

Memory games have each player add another item and the following player must recite the growing list before adding a new item. ("I went on a trip and with me I brought my hat, a guitar, a baby sea turtle, etc…")

There are loads of other games as well that can be played to help you get through a challenging meal. The goal is to distract you from issues of food and calories and all other mealtime concerns *temporarily* in order to get through the meal. That being said, an alphabet category such as "food items" would probably not help very much. Although I will mention that during my time in treatment (and especially towards the end of treatment) I would sit with my friends and play games that all but mocked the situation. Categories included "medication names" and "things that would be taken away if you brought them to treatment." As you can see, we had fun with it, and you can too. Be creative.

These games can help you get through some of the more difficult moments with food, or as a friend of mine calls them, "struggle meals." In order to break free of the eating disorder, you need to get out of the mindset of the eating disorder.

"It takes a while to move into that place," Jodi Krumholz says. "People do feel that once they're working with me they have the permission that they need to eat. That helps to alleviate a little bit of the anxiety. Then it's about consistently coping – counter journaling, etc., until over time the eating disorder voice quiets down."

"When your brain is starving you're not thinking clearly," Jodi continues. "Eating helps in terms of your ability to do therapy, think clearly… Just like any other physical symptom, you cannot recover if your brain is starving. You just can't do the cognitive work that way."

Proper, consistent nutrition also helps you become more able to utilize the support you have in your life. Depending on your specific situation, you may or may not have the support of your family, or whomever you live with, or you may live alone. Jodi admits that a lack of family support presents a formidable challenge.

People need healthy role models of coping in their lives, especially when they are trying to recover from an eating disorder or other addictive illness. "Parents may not cope appropriately," cautions Jodi, "A lot of the way people cope is learned [from their parents]. Parents may not always be good role models."

"Unfortunately," says Jodi, "it's going to be very challenging to get better in this environment." When asked how someone in this situation can recover, Jodi advises, "Use your team as role models. Find other people in your life who are healthier role models, spend more time with healthy friends and relatives."

"Acquire as many support systems as possible for yourself," says Jodi. This is true for everyone; however, it is especially crucial for those with less supportive families.

In recovery we spend a lot of time surrounding ourselves with those who know more than we do in terms of healthy living. We learn from them and try to internalize the messages and lessons we glean from them. We also have to remember that deep inside of us we do have the strength we need to succeed and the knowledge of what is right.

At a certain point I learned to appreciate my own wisdom and choose my own path in life. It took me a while, and in many ways it is still a work in progress, but I am finally becoming what I call "my own home base." Instead of turning to someone else for *answers*, I turn to others for *guidance*. This requires a great deal of honesty and integrity.

Going back to a point made earlier in this book, it is important to recognize and fully accept where you are in your recovery at any given time. Slipping doesn't mean you have relapsed and a relapse doesn't mean your life is over, no matter how much it feels that way. You may slip back into similar struggles, and you may even experience *new* struggles you never had before. Sometimes, in hindsight, you will wonder, "How did I not see this coming?" You might become frustrated with your lack of foresight. It's normal to feel this way, even though it *is* pretty unrealistic. It's always easier to look back and identify warning signs than it is to see them at the time they are happening.

For example, when I was in the very early stages of recovery I wanted absolute, solid reassurance that it was impossible for me to eat too much. I wanted to know that no matter how much I ate it would never become a problem of overeating. In order to allay my fears, my parents told me what I "needed" to hear. And in retrospect it quite possibly *was* what I needed to hear. But I also desperately needed to work on balance. Not too much food, not too little food. Balance.

In residential treatment I became frustrated sometimes with what seemed to be small portion sizes. Of course, I whined and complained about how it was "too much food," because, after all, I had to be that "perfect eating disorder patient." But you know what? Deep down I was truly frustrated because I wanted to eat *more.* People in the general population seem to have this idea that people with eating disorders, especially anorexia, don't like food (or that they like food *too much*!). For me, I loved food. I spent my time thinking about food. I dreaded mealtimes, but I looked forward to them just as much, if not more. Many times, I secretly wanted more food on my plate. I wanted to know that in recovery I would never starve again. I wanted to be full and satisfied. *What I wish someone had told me was that the physical hunger I felt in the depths of my eating disorder was far more intense than anything I would feel in recovery.*

For me, this translated into overeating – something I'd never struggled with prior to my recovery. I overate at restaurants, at parties, and alone at home. I justified it, telling myself, "At least I'm not restricting – it's better to err on the side of eating too much!" I lost track of my hunger and fullness in the opposite direction for a while. Thankfully, once I was honest about my struggles, my therapist taught me a helpful trick to aid in my determination of hunger and fullness. She told me that when people start eating (assuming they are eating mindfully), the food has a stronger taste, and when they start getting full, the food loses a bit of its flavor. That became a sign of fullness for me. Were things perfect from then on out? No. But I was more aware. I still overate on some occasions and I still under-ate on some occasions.

Social worker and registered dietitian Ellyn Satter wrote a wonderful essay demonstrating an ideal relationship with food. This popular essay is often used to teach healthy eating to those who struggle with food:

What is Normal Eating?[1]

Normal eating is going to the table hungry and eating until you are satisfied. It is being able to choose food you like and eat it and truly get enough of it – not just stop eating because you think you should. Normal eating is being able to give some thought to your food selection so you get nutritious food, but not being so wary and restrictive that you miss out on enjoyable food. Normal eating is giving yourself permission to eat sometimes because you are happy, sad or bored, or just because it feels good. Normal eating is mostly three meals a day, or four or five, or it can be choosing to munch along the way. It is leaving some cookies on the plate because you know you can have some again tomorrow, or it is eating more now because they taste so wonderful. Normal eating is overeating at times, feeling stuffed and uncomfortable. And it can be undereating at times and wishing you had more. Normal eating is trusting your body to make up for your mistakes in eating. Normal eating takes up some of your time and attention, but keeps its place as only one important area of your life.

In short, normal eating is flexible. It varies in response to your hunger, your schedule, your proximity to food and your feelings.

---

1   Copyright © 2009 by Ellyn Satter. Published at www.ellynsatter.com.

℘ Jessica

Looking into the mirror used to be the greatest source of distress for Jessica. Nothing she saw ever pleased her. She picked on various parts of her body, her eyes drawn to her "imperfections." Too fat. Too bulky. Too ugly. Her eyes found problems everywhere and demanded she change to accommodate unrealistic strivings for "perfection."

Dieting gave way to rigid calorie-counting obsessions. Jessica had to know exactly what was in her food at all times. She limited her intake, eating less and less. Jessica lost weight and controlling her weight loss became an added addiction. Her health worsened and her thoughts deteriorated into a tangled mess of "not good enough" and "not sick enough." At one point Jessica was terribly distressed because she was not on a feeding tube. If only she needed to be force-fed through a tube she would finally be "sick enough" and be worthy! Worthy of praise, worthy of love, worthy of help.

Then one day Jessica sat beside a mirror and just stared into her eyes – those same eyes that were forever scrutinizing her flaws. For the first time she saw the truth and not the fake smile. She saw the lies, the pain, the hurt, the uncertainty. And worst of all, she saw the emptiness. No longer was Jessica happy, confident, and free spirited. She was fake and empty. A cheap imitation of her former self.

This painful episode served as a wake-up call to Jessica. She had to work at therapy, she had to give it her all. She had to work at her recovery and follow her meal plans and sometimes *just get through it* even when she didn't want to. She had to fight to get her old self back. She *had* to. She couldn't live like this. The process was long and arduous but somewhere in the midst of it all, Jessica caught an occasional glimpse in the mirror. She saw a new set of eyes looking back at her. In those eyes was acceptance – the soul of a girl who could accept change. She saw maturity, she saw desire. And best of all, she saw life. The road had not been easy but there was no sign of fakeness in those eyes. Life had returned to the Jessica within.

Chapter 6

ACCEPTING YOUR BODY

"Most of the shadows of this life are caused
by standing in one's own sunshine."

– Ralph Waldo Emerson

A year and a half into my recovery I spent a week in Florida visiting friends and making plans for graduate school. One evening after dinner, a friend's father turned to me and said, "I know you have some kind of eating disorder, but you've been here for a week and I have no idea what the problem is." I explained to him that I am in recovery and am no longer engaging in symptoms.

"May I ask what kind of eating disorder you had?" he questioned.

"Anorexia," I told him.

An expression of disbelief appeared on his face. He looked me up and down and said incredulously, "*You* were *anorexic*? Well *boy* did *you* recover!"

My friend's father had never before interacted with anyone he knew to have an eating disorder. He meant well but did not know the "right" things to say. As for me, I found it to be one of the funniest comments I'd ever heard in recovery but I also realized that it had the potential to cause untold anxiety to those currently struggling with their eating disorders. I explained to him that it's not possible to know if a person has an eating disorder based on looks alone. Many people suffering from eating disorders appear healthy. Comments about appearance in relation to eating disorders can be especially harmful when a person is struggling to seek treatment. Many are hesitant to ask for help when they don't think they look sick enough to warrant treatment. Furthermore, those advancing in recovery often fear looking better before feeling better – as if their outward appearance is their only avenue of communicating their pain.

The idea that someone with an eating disorder must look a certain way is an offshoot of a dangerous misconception rooted deeply in today's looks-focused society – the way something looks must be the way it is.

Jessica

Jessica was recruited to play college softball during the early stages of her eating disorder. She was supposed to be a power-hitter but because she didn't allow herself adequate nutrition she was unable to play her part. Her coach told her that because she was physically smaller than most other girls on the team she should also be faster. Jessica had an idea of what the fast girls looked like and she began dieting and over-exercising in order to match that image.

As she spiraled deeper into her eating disorder, Jessica was in grave danger. Her parents and treatment team made arrangements for her to enter a women's residential treatment facility. On her first day Jessica was horrified by the other patients. The first woman she met looked so sick and emaciated. *I'm not small enough to be here*, Jessica worried as the patient hugged her. Later in the day Jessica met an average-sized girl who had been in treatment for over two months. She had curly blond hair, blue eyes, and a huge smile. She was the most beautiful girl that Jessica had ever seen. Yet rather than inspiring hope, a crushing feeling of inadequacy overcame Jessica as she told herself, *I can't live up to either girl – healthy or sick.*

Upon entering treatment for her eating disorder Jessica was unable to distinguish between her body image and her identity. She felt that she had two choices – play the role in which her perceived body image cast her or change her appearance to fit a new role.

When a person has an eating disorder the boundaries between body image and identity are often blurred. The longer a person remains entrenched in an eating disorder, the harder it is to make that important distinction. This is one reason why it is important to take action – to find a treatment team, work hard, and develop and strengthen healthy coping skills – as soon as possible when you suspect an eating disorder or when you are in recovery but starting to slip.

One of the most important skills to develop in order to help differentiate between your body image and yourself is the ability to express yourself in new and healthy ways. Specific methods of creative expression will be discussed in Chapter 7; however, the underlying theme uniting all of them is the need for a healthy outlet and manner of communication. Using your voice – learning to express your needs and feelings verbally – is the best way to begin moving away from using your body to communicate your messages.

Social worker and trauma specialist Regina Lukens often tells her clients that having an eating disorder is a way to "fight back." Hurting yourself is a way to hurt those who love and care about you. Eating disorders are sometimes an attempt to tell people "I'm not okay – look what you did to me." A recovery friend of mine once reminded me, "Your family doesn't speak Eating-Disorder. Use your words."

Regina teaches her clients that giving up the eating disorder is *not* tantamount to giving up the fight. Recovery is not defeat and it is not giving up.

 ## Taylor

Taylor's eating disorder was originally a frantic attempt to get attention and care from her father. It spiraled into an all-out war against her family. And finally, it became an identity. For a long time, Taylor felt like recovery meant giving up a part of herself. It meant conceding and throwing in the towel. But in reality, Taylor's recovery provided just the opposite.

"Recovery was actually empowering, even in the beginning," Taylor reminisces. It meant that she found new ways of getting her needs met that actually *worked*. Whereas the eating disorder didn't help people "get it" in regards to what she needed, recovery enabled her to take a more direct approach. When she needed validation, for example, she was able to outright *ask* for exactly what she needed. Sometimes it was as specific as telling a co-worker, "I need you to tell me that I did well on this project."

While still in her eating disorder days, Taylor was unable to seek out what she needed, even when she *knew* what she needed. This led to feelings of frustration and inadequacy, compounding her already dismal self-esteem. When asked if she took her feelings out on her body, Taylor responded, "Oh yes, all the freaking time!" Taylor felt so horribly about herself. In an eating disordered effort to make her insides match her outsides, Taylor did horrible things *to* herself in order to get other people to understand how she was feeling.

"It's really not an issue anymore today," she says. "I guess a part of it was learning to validate things for myself. And learning that it is much more effective to *tell* someone how I'm doing than to *show* them."

Recovery was still a difficult process to begin. Taylor recalls that initially she resigned herself to the thought that, "Okay, I'm just going to have to be fat. So what." It was hard for her to think outside of a black-and-white box and it took her a long time to get there.

"It's still hard for me sometimes. But now it's hard in other ways. It's not just about my body – it's about my whole self. I feel like I need to constantly be improving myself. Changing my body gave me an easy way to get that feeling, even though it wasn't real. Sometimes it's still hard to fully grasp that, but in time things have gotten much better."

Negative body image is painful and can often feed into an eating disorder. However, to say that negative body image *causes* eating disorders is largely inaccurate, although the statement does retain some credibility. A popular theory in the field of psychology, called the "diathesis stress model," claims that a person is born with a certain genetic predisposition to various disorders – such as depression and eating disorders – but that the disorders lie dormant until they are triggered by an environmental factor. According to this model it makes sense that a person with negative body image who simply "goes on a diet" in order to lose weight may run into trouble, as the diet itself may bring about the onset of an eating disorder. Dieting, more than exercising, is suspected to trigger eating disorders in some people. In fact, this is one proposed reason for the incidence of eating disorders being higher in women than in men: Women are more likely to diet when they wish to lose weight, while men are more likely to exercise. Nevertheless, poor body image does not directly *cause* eating disorders. Eating disorders are far too complicated to be blamed on any one cause, or even a number of causes.

The longer the eating disorder-body image distortion cycle continues, the harder it is to find yourself and to break free. The disorder itself can become a game in which the sicker you are, the more points you earn. The good news is that you make your own rules in this game and you can change them...

When I was still very entrenched in my eating disorder I got rid of all the clothing that fit me when I was healthy. I was convinced that I would never be so "big" again and therefore I would never fit into those clothes again. When I came home from residential treatment, my mother helped me go through and give away my "sick clothes" that no longer fit. I was left without any jeans.

"Why did you get rid of all your healthy-sized pants?" my mother asked me.

"I thought I'd never wear them again. They were the wrong size," I said.

She replied, "Did you ever stop to think that maybe your *pants* were the right size and *you* weren't?"

The message was clear. Struggling doesn't mean you have to give up hope of someday recovering. For me, it was a bit more complicated than my mother realized. Back when I was sick I had been playing an "eating disorder game" in which I got rid of my larger clothing to prevent myself from ever fitting into them again. I looked at the clothing that fit me when I was healthy in astonishment and disgust that they *ever* fit me and vowed that they never would again.

Nonetheless, my mother was right. I would have been better off had I put the clothes away somewhere rather than dump them completely. The game I played with my clothes when I was sick only served to make me sicker. In true eating disorder form, I had boxed myself into another set of rules: I had to keep my body dimensions exactly as they were – or smaller. I had to be able to wear those same clothes forever. If I didn't, that meant I was a failure. A *fat* failure.

If you are going through a similar struggle, you may identify with this mindset. The recovery process can be terrifying. There were times during my treatment when well-meaning friends and family members would tell me that *they* didn't starve themselves, did I think they were fat? I always answered no because I didn't want to hurt them. But inside there was a raging torrent of "YES! I think you are a cow and I'd rather have an eating disorder forever than look like you!" I even wrote in my journal at one point that I was happy when other people recover from eating disorders because then there was less competition to be the smallest.

Fast-forward to a day over two years into my recovery. I went shopping with my family to buy formal clothing for a new job. A saleswoman helped me find new outfits and began by asking me my pants size. I gladly told her. It was nothing personal. The number no longer represented to me my value or self-worth. At another store I tried on a pair of jeans that clearly stated on the tag, "curvy fit." When they fit me, I felt a bit of pride. I am happy and healthy and this is my body. I may not like everything about it all the time, but it is part of who I am and I love it. Perhaps the most important thing is that negative body image no longer dictates my mood or my actions regarding food and exercise.

So how does such a transformation take place?

Jessica

For Jessica, body acceptance began with an abstract exercise in her therapist's office in which she pinpointed perceived "problem areas" on her body and assigned each of them a different color. Her head was "too big" and Jessica assigned it the color black. Her legs, about which she was self-conscious, were brown. Her stomach was a dirty, dark gray color. Jessica also identified a positive – her heart – and assigned it the color orange. She couldn't quite explain why, since she's "not a huge fan of orange," but the color was safe and calming.

Going through each body part and assigning it a color was an uncomfortable experience for Jessica. She didn't just name body parts and colors, but rather she and her therapist discussed each pair. Her "brown legs" were a point of discomfort, for example, because when she was fourteen years old her mother told her that she had "football player legs." Jessica was an athletic teenager but that comment made her wonder if she should stop working out. She cried as she recalled negative comments made by her grandmother when she was nine years old. Her grandmother used to pat Jessica's stomach and tell her that she was a "full-figured girl" and that she "obviously doesn't care what she eats." Jessica didn't like to be touched then and she still doesn't. To this day Jessica hates having her stomach touched as it reminds her of the self-disgust she felt as a child upon hearing her grandmother's criticism of her body.

At times the exercise overwhelmed Jessica. She felt ashamed of "telling on her family" and she had memories of physical pain so intense she had to take breaks. Her therapist worked at Jessica's pace, gently guiding her. The therapist also helped Jessica to sit still and avoid numbing her feelings through movements, especially shaking her leg – a common numbing behavior among those with eating disorders. After naming colors for every troubling body part and exploring the connections in her past, Jessica felt a greater understanding. She also felt more united with her body, grounded. It was as though a weight was lifted from her and she could begin to move towards self-acceptance.

Jessica also benefitted from affirmations which helped to counter the negative messages she received in her younger years. After years of being referred to as an "ugly duckling" by friends and family, Jessica came to believe she was unattractive. When we are constantly flooded with any type of messages we can come to believe them. The good news is that we can later reject negative messages and replace them with positive ones. Jessica never lied to herself, but rather made statements of fact, such as:

"I do not have cankles."

"If seeing bones stick out on other people isn't attractive, then it isn't attractive on me either."

"My weight does not determine my happiness."

We always have the ability to rewrite the scripts playing through our minds. Affirmations sometimes start off as superficial statements about body image, but they can develop into genuine declarations of self-worth and purpose.

Lexi

There was a time when Lexi could not even pass by a mirror without staring at it in disappointment. Every mirror seemed to speak to her – words of hopelessness, hatred, and despair. During the dark days of her eating disorder, nothing about Lexi's appearance satisfied her. Even her eyes and her smile, things Lexi used to like, didn't please her anymore. It wasn't only her distorted body image coming into play – it was who the eating disorder was making her. Her eyes were dead, her smile fake.

Lexi's therapist suggested she cover her bathroom mirror, leaving only enough room for her face. Lexi covered over the mirror with different colored paper. On the paper she wrote down things she liked about herself. Not physical things, but rather personality traits. She also included a few quotes and Bible verses she found inspiring. The goal was to remind Lexi that there was more to her than her looks. Every morning Lexi saw the words on her mirror and even if she wasn't yet ready or able to see anything positive in her reflection, the words on the mirror began to help her see the good.

One morning Lexi noticed that next to an affirmation stating "good sister," her brother had written, "yep!" She wonders if her brother will ever understand how much his simple validation meant to her during such a difficult time. As Lexi began to seek out the positive qualities in herself, and to accept that others can see them too, her body image slowly improved. She is more than her weight, her body, and her looks. She is a full person, capable of tremendous good. She is loved by her family and friends. She is beautiful.

Lexi still has days when it is difficult to draw her focus away from physical characteristics that trouble her. On those days, Lexi consciously reminds herself that she is beautiful in God's eyes and that she was created with a purpose much deeper than the image she sees in the mirror.

One of the most helpful lessons I have learned in recovery is that the real world doesn't function in black and white, but rather in shades of gray… and purple and orange and sometimes even in colors that glitter and glow in the dark. You can't choose what comes your way and you can't plan for all of it either. You *can* however, choose not to take it out on your body. This isn't always easy. I have found that no matter how positive my body image may be on any given day, there are still days when it feels hopeless. That's when it comes in handy to remember that life isn't black and white. Hopelessness itself isn't always a bad thing, and like any challenge, it can be channeled and used to your benefit.

Dr. Mark Warren of the Cleveland Center for Eating Disorders helps his clients attain a more positive body image through realistic affirmations. Many people entering treatment expect to be prescribed the classic "affirmations," looking in the mirror and telling themselves nice things about their bodies until they believe them. These types of instructions discourage a lot of people who don't understand how outright lying to their reflections in the mirror is going to help. If you are one of those people, there is hope. Dr. Warren never asks people to blatantly lie to themselves.

"Don't tell yourself you like something you don't," he says, "instead, work on acceptance." Accepting a body whose image you associate with tremendous struggling is admittedly very difficult and may take a long time. Dr. Warren recommends affirmations as a way to develop and enhance this much-needed acceptance. The first step is simply telling yourself, "This is my body. This is it – the only body I get. Accept it. I must find a way." And this is where some channeled hopelessness can ease the way.

When I think of the body shape and size I sometimes wish to have, the body I want when I am experiencing a particularly difficult challenge, I remind myself of a simple biological fact: My body is built a certain way and there is no way to change that. Diet and exercise cannot spot-reduce perceived "problem areas." No matter how much or how little a person weighs, the body will retain a certain proportion. In this sense, it is "hopeless."

People with eating disorders strive to impact and change their bodies' appearances, often with disappointing results. Sometimes the eating disorder gets in the way of their efforts and sometimes they are just not satisfied with their "accomplishments." When I was in the depths of my eating disorder I wanted more than anything to reach a certain number on the scale. I still remember the moment I stepped on the scale and saw the number. I thought I would be ecstatic, but instead I just felt hungry and tired and sick. The only thought I had was a desperate *that's it*?! I didn't feel the sense of completion and contentment because there is no such thing in the eating disordered mind as "thin enough" or "good enough." I always wanted more, more, more.

During moments of disappointing body image in my recovery, these memories bring about a *healthy hopelessness* which reminds me that no matter how strongly I believe in this current moment that losing a few pounds or attempting to change my body in any given way will bring me satisfaction, it is nothing but an illusion. Not only that, but during these moments my feelings about my body would be negative at any weight! It is hopeless to try to change my body to reach an unattainable goal.

It may feel unpleasant in the moment, but refusing to sabotage your recovery has immense rewards later on. This moment may feel unpleasant but acting on it will only perpetuate the pain. Each time you refuse to engage in symptoms to satisfy a momentary urge, you strengthen your belief in a better future.

Korrie

The summer before her fourth grade year, Korrie looked in the mirror at sleep-away camp and saw an image of a fat girl. She began complaining about how fat she was, even though her weight was normal. Everyone around her thought she was doing it for attention. In gymnastics she would suck in her stomach, telling her coach that she did it because she was fat. By seventh grade Korrie felt depressed and inadequate. She believed that if only she changed her appearance she would be treated differently by her peers and by people in general. She joined Weight Watchers with her mother and began losing weight. Much to Korrie's delight, people *did* treat her differently. Weight loss was seemingly rewarded and these new feelings of accomplishment and acceptance reinforced Korrie's beliefs that dieting was the solution to all of her problems.

Unfortunately this euphoria was accompanied by illness. Mentally and physically, Korrie took a turn for the worse. She was hospitalized on numerous occasions and was admitted to a psychiatric ward following a planned suicide attempt. Once again, Korrie was miserable.

After a lot of hard work and treatment, including inpatient and residential stays, Korrie achieved a basic level of recovery. She minimized her use of symptoms and learned to express herself in healthier ways. Korrie realized that no matter what size she was, she was never happy. She acknowledged that all of the time she spent on changing her appearance could be used towards being happy and she'd be better off for it. Even in more advanced stages of recovery, she explains, it still sounds much easier than it actually is. In addition, her body image did not significantly improve, which was continually a source of distress and frustration.

At a certain point Korrie had been in recovery but struggling for a while. She went to her therapist and cried for the first time. For the first time she was talking about *herself*. Not about other people and drama and things that didn't matter. Korrie was finally getting in touch with her emotions. In a moment of blazing clarity she realized that she'd been waiting for her parents, friends – *everyone* – to change. But she finally understood, in that moment, that it wasn't about any of them. It was about her. Korrie. If she wanted to be happier, then *she* was the one who needed to change. It was hard because Korrie didn't like to admit that anything was her fault or her responsibility.

The more time Korrie spent talking about herself in therapy, the more she realized that her outer appearance wasn't the issue. The real issue was that she was hurting inside and didn't want to deal with it. Subconsciously, Korrie hid from her real problems and covered them up with the eating disorder.

"When you compare yourself to other people," she says, "you realize that there are always people who you think are thinner than you, bigger than you, prettier than you. And in the end all you get is a feeling of inadequacy and worthlessness." Korrie also shares the following hard-earned wisdom:

"When I have bad body image it feels bad, but I don't have to give in to it. I used to like bad body image because it meant I could act on my symptoms. Now I sit through it. It's still hard, but I get through it. The most rewarding feeling is to actually like myself. Even if it's only for a day – or even if it's only for five minutes. It gives me hope that I can make it more long term."

Perhaps the greatest catalyst for making peace with my body was learning to appreciate my body for what it can do rather than for how it looks. This is a slow process with many ups and downs. The first positive body image moment I remember was during my time at Renfrew. I was sitting in a large armchair during a group therapy session and suddenly became aware that my body was not as painfully thin as it had been previously. I was able to cuddle up in the chair contentedly and the sensation comforted me.

That isn't to say that it was smooth sailing from then on because that most certainly was not the case. As time went on, however, the positive moments grew stronger and more frequent and it became easier for me to cope with the negative moments.

One of the most important lessons I learned in treatment is that not every struggle must be dealt with in depth in the moment. Sometimes it is okay to let things go for a period of time and come back to them later. Containment writing, which will be discussed in Chapter 7, is an excellent way to put things on the backburner until you can fully deal with them at a more appropriate time. This enables you to continue to function in the present moment and can be especially helpful at mealtimes. If, for example, you feel too "fat" to eat – or too depressed or too anxious – then a simple distraction can be helpful in getting you through a meal. Play a word game, practice mindfulness skills, talk to others at the table about things not related to food or body image. Some suggestions can be found in Chapter 5.

The same concept of distraction holds true for a variety of different situations. Sometimes you will not be able to resolve your negative body image, at least not in the moment. Sometimes you will feel negatively about your body and you will need to just manage and cope with it. Discovering the meaning behind your body image may help you feel better about yourself, as sometimes negative body image symbolizes a deeper struggle. If there truly are deeper issues involved then it is definitely worth exploring them with a qualified therapist. However, sometimes body image really is just a surface issue.

Body image is a struggle for many, including those without eating disorders. Although I always knew this on some level, I understood it more deeply during an appointment with my nutritionist.

"I feel fat," I tearfully told her one afternoon. I'd been feeling strong and positive for a while and this sudden, intense concern was somewhat out of the blue for me.

"What brought this on?" my nutritionist asked me.

"I went shopping for a bathing suit yesterday and I tried on so many of them and none of them fit right!"

"Naomi," she said, "you are a woman and women often have trouble finding flattering bathing suits. Women dealing with eating disorders often think they are the only ones who have a hard time shopping for swimsuits or jeans, but it's not true – *almost everyone* shares these issues, eating disorder or not!"

It was something to think about and even though I fought her in the moment, ("yeah, but it's not the *same!*") I soon came to realize that she was right. I spoke with my mother and sister about their body image concerns. They both also have to find clothing that accommodates their bodies' shapes and sizes. In speaking with my sister I discovered a crucial difference. While she seeks to find *clothing* that fits her *body*, during my eating disorder days I sought to make my *body* fit the *clothing*. My sister knows that her body image has nothing to do with her worth or value. When she came home at the end of a study abroad program having gained a bit of weight, she simply carried on with her life and let her weight drift back to its original set-point naturally. She admittedly wasn't thrilled about the gain, but she also didn't let it cramp her style. It brought to mind a comment made by a friend's younger brother during a multi-family therapy group at the Renfrew Center.

"If the shirt you tried on doesn't fit," he said innocently, "don't change yourself – just get a bigger shirt!" His advice generated a bit of laughter from the patients and families in the room dealing with eating disorders, but he was on to something important: Why change ourselves to fit an artificial mold when we can respect and appreciate ourselves the way we are meant to be?

Andrew

"I was afraid of anyone seeing me for who I was," says Andrew. "I thought I was a terrible person. I don't know why. I remember feeling worthless, like a burden, like I had nothing to contribute for as long as I can remember. And that's despite having really good parents who did as much for me as they possibly could."

A major part of Andrew's recovery was to change his beliefs about himself. Andrew felt like he would be alone for the rest of his life. He didn't associate with anybody, so in effect he was *keeping* himself alone. The eating disorder was a way for Andrew to numb out and block away the painful feelings of inadequacy that plagued him incessantly. He spent all of his time wrapped up in eating disorder thoughts and behaviors, leaving little to no time to think about anything else or anybody else. It kept him from ruminating about how he hated himself.

Therapy, over time, was the biggest contributor to Andrew's recovery. Care working with Stephanie helped as well.

"They got me to see the irrationalness of my thoughts. When I saw that, I was willing to change. I was being irrational about me being a bad person. [Other] people aren't judging me and thinking I'm a bad person."

Now Andrew says that he suspects everyone has days when they feel bad about themselves. Even after recovery.

"But not to the extent that you would hurt yourself or be destructive," he clarifies.

Whether you feel bad about yourself or your body, everyone has days like that.

"I suppose it depends on how much emphasis you put on your appearance," says Andrew. "We're more than a body. Our bodies are a very small part of who we are. I think striving for perfection is a common characteristic in eating disorders. If you let go of it, then it becomes perfectly okay to have bad body image days."

According to Rebekah Bardwell Doweyko, reacting negatively to poor body image is often a matter of control. "It's much easier to say 'I feel fat' than 'I feel scared' or 'I feel anxious' or 'I feel angry,'" she says. For many people who feel out of control emotionally, changing their bodies becomes an avenue to take charge. "Feelings are more ambiguous," says Rebekah, "You can't see them. You can't measure them... You have to make yourself vulnerable in order to talk about [feelings]. When you say things like, 'I feel fat,' you're not sharing any sort of internal struggle. You're just looking for people to say, 'Oh no you're not – you're beautiful!' You know you'll get some response that is in no way challenging." Rebekah says that instead of simply looking in the mirror and just seeing the body, people should introspect and also see their intrinsic qualities. When you look in the mirror, think about your true self. Think about those things that make you who you are. "Our bodies are just our shells," says Rebekah. Use yours to live the best life you can.

 ## Aurora

A turning point in the quality of Aurora's self-concept came after her therapist shared with her the wisdom of Alanis Morissette who advises people to treat their bodies as instruments rather than as ornaments. The therapist also suggested that Aurora thank her body for its functions that she had previously taken for granted. Aurora took these lessons to heart and began thanking her body for the things it did for her:

"I thank my eyes for seeing."

"I thank my lungs for breathing."

"I thank my hands for writing."

It was this last expression of gratitude that eventually led to a breakthrough. After years of practice and perseverance, Aurora came to appreciate that her body's weight and appearance were insignificant compared to its function as the instrument of her creativity.

Although Aurora had always been artistically inclined, her art and writing took on new meaning and purpose as she advanced in her recovery. She founded a recovery-oriented organization aimed at helping women empower themselves through self-expression and creativity. Promoting this cause became more than a passion for Aurora – it was a calling. Through years of her own treatment, Aurora had learned the value of creative expression. She recognized that creativity and the synchronization of body, mind, and soul went hand in hand.

Getting to this point isn't an easy task. Even in recovery there are levels of success and times when success comes easier than at other times. Connecting body, mind, and soul is a challenge for anyone and it is a stage of recovery that usually comes after the initial health-stabilization period. Even then Aurora says, "It takes a lot of practice and it's something I'm still working on."

Aurora is not completely symptom-free, but she is working towards a day when she will be. There are still days when maintaining a healthy lifestyle is difficult. Sometimes body image presents a formidable challenge. But through her struggles for higher levels of recovery and for increasing development and growth, Aurora is discovering that she is capable of things far beyond her physical appearance. She can give. She can empower. She can create. Her body is the instrument – and she is the musician.

Chapter 7

GETTING CREATIVE

"Let yourself live the life you were
once capable of living."

– Jessica

Almost two years into my recovery I began working with the Renfrew Center on a series of programs called "Rewriting Our Stories." Each event, geared primarily toward former patients and members of the community, is an opportunity for participants to explore their life stories and to empower themselves to make whatever changes are necessary for them to live the lives they choose. This is done through several creative workshops comprised of activities such as writing, movement, and art.

People come to these events in varying situations. Some of the participants come in need of further treatment. Some are struggling a bit. Some are maintaining a solid state of recovery. What is interesting to note is that people at all stages have connected with the workshops and done meaningful work. There is no point in a struggle when recovery exercises are hopeless and there is no point in recovery when recovery exercises are pointless. They are never beyond you and you are never beyond them.

Honest self-expression

Eating disorders keep things inside and allow them to cause pain by surfacing in unhealthy ways. Recovery helps break the cycle. Self-expression is a key component to a healthy life. It is important to recognize and accept where you are at any given moment and to express yourself honestly.

When I was thirteen years old I was hurting. I was angry with my family and school and friends. I was extremely depressed and wanted help but didn't know how to express myself or how to get what I needed. I thought that if I outright asked for support no one would take me seriously. I thought that asking for help meant no one would give me what I needed and I'd wind up feeling worse than before. I mistakenly believed that others would think that since I was able to ask for help, I wasn't really so bad off. In my mind the only solution was to act out my misery. I engaged in unhealthy behaviors and cried a lot. I thought that I had to always be unhappy or else no one would know I was hurting and no one would help me. I thought I could never smile or be happy because that would mean I didn't really need help.

The same thoughts played out in many different situations, not the least of which was the eating disorder I developed a short while later. It took me until I was twenty years old – and in recovery – to recognize the error in my thinking. After eleven weeks in residential treatment I came to understand that speaking up gets my needs met and understood in a much more efficient and real way than acting out.

It wasn't an easy lesson in the least. You may be familiar with the phenomenon of eating disorder patients who don't think they are – or look – "sick enough" to warrant treatment. It's the same idea. As I went through treatment I learned to give voice to my hurt. My *voice* became the instrument I used to let people know when I was hurting, when I was frustrated, when I was angry, and so on. Not my *body*.

I also learned that just because I was struggling, that didn't mean I couldn't have a good day. Smiling, laughing, and enjoying the company of others did not mean I didn't deserve help. Conversely, after I reached a solid state of recovery, that didn't mean I couldn't have a bad day and express struggles. Everyone has struggles – eating disorder history or not. It's not about the struggle, but rather about how you choose to cope with it. It *is* a choice.

Use your voice. You have probably heard this phrase more times than you care to count. Speaking up and voicing your needs is certainly an important skill, however, not all voice is verbal. How do you best express yourself? Do you connect with art or music? What about movement or writing? These are all healthy ways to explore and discover what lies beneath the surface and help your thoughts and feelings find much needed expression.

Writing

Putting thoughts and feelings into words is a skill that can be learned just like any other. There are many ways to use writing to your benefit at all stages of recovery. The same exercises can be used for different purposes or modified to help you achieve specific recovery – or life – goals.

Letter-writing exercises

Shortly before I sought treatment for my eating disorder at age twenty I was studying abroad in Israel. At my lowest point I had become very ill and rarely left my bed. I received some outpatient care as a young teenager and maintained a sort of quasi-recovery for a few years but because I hadn't been in intensive treatment before, I didn't know very much about formal recovery exercises. Even the word "recovery" was foreign to me. I wasn't convinced I had an eating disorder but I knew that I wasn't well. One night I wrote a letter to my future self. It was a way for me to express my pain while at the same time mentally draw on my future strength and discourage myself from ever relapsing once I found recovery. The letter has since been lost, but here is a partial recreation:

Dear Naomi,

It is the middle of the night and I cannot sleep. I am hungry and exhausted but I cannot eat. I am completely miserable. I want you to remember this moment in case you ever find yourself thinking life will be better if only you lose weight. It will only lead you down this path of misery once again. The "good" moments when someone compliments your appearance or when you reach a lower number on the scale pale in comparison to the bad moments when you are all alone, starving and weak, consumed with thoughts of food and numbers. There are no answers in starvation and there is no peace or happiness. You will not feel better about your body or yourself. (The letter then goes on to detail my body image complaints at my lowest weight.) *I started writing this letter in order to support you, but really it is me who needs the support. I feel trapped. You know happiness and life. You are not bound by diets and self-hatred. I will draw on your strength because you have already made it through to the other side. And ultimately, that means so will I.*

Love, Naomi

The letter helped me imagine a time when I could be free from my eating disorder. The last line is especially important. I envisioned myself "winning the race," so to speak. Later on many people would ask me if at my lowest point I could ever have imagined recovery. I tell them honestly, "yes." The moment I wrote this letter I knew I would get better. I didn't know when or how, but I knew it would happen because I *wanted* it and I *believed* it would happen.

It was still several months before I found the help I needed in residential treatment. Even then I wanted to recover but not gain any weight (which for me was impossible). Recovery has been a long and often challenging journey, but when I wrote this letter I knew that somehow I would make it. It was my very first baby step toward healing.

If you are struggling to find motivation you may find this particular exercise helpful. Begin by imagining your future self. Who are you? What are you doing? What does your life look like? Remember, your future self can be anything you choose. It is a reflection of your hopes and dreams. Write a letter drawing on those qualities you wish to have. Make your future self a concrete entity. And know that everything that person has done, by definition you can and will do too.

Another letter-writing exercise involves writing a letter from your body to yourself. An example of this can be found in my first book, *One Life*. The idea behind this type of letter is to help you think about yourself in a new light. If your body could talk, what would it say? What would it say specifically to *you*?

This exercise can be adapted in many ways. You might try writing a letter to your eating disorder – or from your eating disorder to yourself. Letter-writing can help you explore relationships with other people as well. Some of these letters you may choose to send while other letters you may keep or even destroy.

I have found letter-writing to be immensely helpful in my recovery. Sometimes when I feel I can't quite bring myself to journal in the traditional sense, I write my journal entry as a letter or even an email. I address the letter to someone I trust who I believe cares about me. As I write the letter I imagine that person's care and comforting responses. There have been many times when I ultimately chose to send the letter, or at least to share its contents with a trusted friend, family member, or therapist.

 ## Jessica

As a part of her relapse-prevention planning at the end of residential treatment, Jessica wrote a letter to herself. She called it her "Rainy Day Letter" and it was from her healthy self to her struggling self. She still reads it during challenging moments and draws strength from it:

> *Dear Struggling Jessica,*
>
> *You can do this. Do not give in because it's not worth it. Remember all the hard work you've put into your recovery. Go to the healthy coping tools: read, pray, counter-journal, talk to someone, Facebook, knit, watch TV, play Wii, go for a drive, play with Squirt (my puppy), go to a movie – just don't give in. You are strong and beautiful. It's okay to feel your feelings. You cannot always be superman. Cry if you want to. Don't shut people out. Be open to feedback. Getting defensive means that you have something to be defensive about. Ask for help. Trust that your support system will not judge you for your thoughts or actions. They are concerned about you and want to help you [even if sometimes they may not know how]. Be patient and hold on to recovery. You deserve a better life than your eating disorder can offer. People really do care so much about you – Jenny, Susan, Tara, Kendra, Mindy, and so many other people who have no idea about anorexia. This is so hard to hear, but "this too shall pass." Your appearance does not define who you are. You have so much to offer to the world and you want to help*

people. You will not be able to help anyone until you can help yourself. You have to get all of you back to live out your dreams. The negative thoughts you have are coming directly from Satan. God has such a better plan for you than what your eating disorder has to offer. Giving in just once leads to compromising later. You are human and therefore you will slip up. Just don't beat yourself to the ground. Get back up and stay strong. Let yourself live the life you were once capable of living. You deserve recovery and will persevere through hard times and struggles. I believe in you and love you just the way you are. DO NOT GIVE UP!

Love Healthy Jessica

Journaling

Free-writing about your day or even about your thoughts and feelings is not the only way to journal. There are many different methods of journaling and many ways to benefit from each of them. Three especially useful techniques are thought records, pro-con lists, and containment writing.

THOUGHT RECORDS

Rebekah Bardwell Doweyko, director and founder of the Center for Intuitive Eating, developed a form of counter journaling called a "thought record" based on the work of cognitive psychologist Aaron Beck. The thought record is designed to help people combat cognitive distortions and challenge their unhealthy and unhelpful thoughts.

Oftentimes people believe that certain thoughts and feelings are "automatic" – that they instantly result from certain external stimuli. This is especially true in the case of eating disorders. Maybe you think that your eating disorder behaviors and urges are an automatic reaction to stress. Maybe you think that becoming angry and blowing up at your family is an automatic response to your frustration with their actions. The idea that feelings are a direct result of the things that happen to us is a misconception. Our feelings are based on our thoughts, and thoughts can be challenged and changed. Even if you have been steeped in an eating disorder or other destructive behavioral pattern for years, there is still a split second of choice. Completing thought records can help you discover the moment between what happens and how you feel – the moment in which you *choose* your response.

Thought records are best completed in the moment, as soon after the distressing incident as possible:

1. Record the event or external stimulus that prompted your distress.

2. Record your feelings about the event.

3. Record your automatic thoughts.

4. Record evidence that supports your thoughts.

5. Record evidence that does not support your thoughts.

6. Record alternate, balanced thoughts.

7. Record feelings again.

It is a good idea to physically write down your thought records and keep them for a while. By completing several thought records you will not only challenge your distorted automatic thoughts, but you will also discover certain patterns. Perhaps you feel resentful when friends ask for favors or scared in new situations or jealous when others receive more attention than you. Once you know your patterns you will be in a better position to counter your "automatic" thoughts with alternate, balanced thoughts.

Discovering these patterns can sometimes be difficult, especially if you think you "shouldn't" feel a certain way. If that is the case, it may be helpful to remind yourself that there is no right way to think or feel. When you don't suppress unwanted feelings – but rather express them in healthy ways – they will be less likely to surface in unhealthy ways.

Sometimes just sitting down and writing can help you find a more balanced perspective. If you are anxious, scared, angry, or frustrated, having something to physically *do* can feel helpful. The time that elapses while you write your thought record can give a little added perspective, giving you a clearer standpoint from which to respond. You do not have control over everything that happens in your life, but you always have choices. Keeping a thought record can help you find them.

Pro-con lists

Pro-con lists are pretty self-explanatory, but there are a couple of variations worth mentioning. The first is obviously to aid the decision-making process by listing all the positive points of one possible decision and weighing them against all the negative points. Pro-con lists can be used not only to make a decision, but also to imagine the future outcomes of different choices.

A worksheet used by the Cleveland Center for Eating Disorders asks clients to imagine their lives in five years with and without their eating disorders. First they are to record how their lives will be in five years without their eating disorder – all the things they can do and achieve in recovery. Then they are to write on the other side of the sheet how their lives will be if they keep their eating disorders. It is a powerful assignment that helps clients think outside of the here and now and into the future to the fulfilling lives they can lead in recovery.

Lexi

"If I were to turn back to my eating disorder today, it might start off as a 'just for today' excuse. I have learned from other relapses that 'just today' is never the case. If in five years I still had my eating disorder, my life would be entirely different than I imagine it will be. First and foremost, I would not be a physical therapist. I would not have the physical or emotional strength to take care of myself much less to hold onto, lift, or help others. I'm sure I would still have some friends but I would be isolating myself from them. Some would give me a tough love ultimatum, trying to get me to see my potential and where my life was, or rather wasn't, going. My family would be so upset every day as they watched me fall apart physically and emotionally, knowing that they could not control me or my choices but wishing they could. I would not have a husband or a family. There is no way I could form a relationship with someone if I was so inwardly focused. My relationship with God would be closed off, by me, not by Him. All of this is if I was alive. There's always the chance that my body could not handle five more years of an eating disorder.

Looking at my life five years from now *without* my eating disorder is a much prettier picture with much more color and life, excitement and joy, love and compassion. I will be using my gifts as a physical therapist, helping others heal and accomplish their goals. My relationships with friends will be real and deep. Maybe I'll even be dating someone or be married. I probably will not have kids yet, but might be thinking about having them. I'm sure my mom will be asking when she's going to get a grandkid though! My life will be full. I will find pleasure in the little blessings of life. I will have energy to run. My thoughts will not be consumed with food or lies but instead, well, I don't know what my thoughts will be – the opportunities are endless! Life without my eating disorder will truly be LIFE."

CONTAINMENT WRITING

Containment is an important skill. Whether you are coping with difficult events in your past or developing healthy boundaries, containment writing is a tool that can aid your progress. For this you will need a containment book and there are different ways to go about choosing one.

At the Renfrew Center patients are often presented with handmade containment books consisting of oversized, unlined sheets of paper. There is another type of containment book, which can simply be a pocket-sized, store-bought notebook. Each of these books can serve as a springboard for successful skill-development.

The purpose of the large books used at Renfrew is to help patients contain their difficult thoughts, feelings, and urges between therapy sessions. This type of book is large enough to accommodate writings, drawings, collages, photos, and whatever else can fit inside those pages. (For three dimensional items, patients use a similarly-themed containment box.)

A smaller book can be used to contain incessant thoughts that might otherwise cause distress or come blurting out at inappropriate times. Many people struggle with their internal "filters" at times, myself included. I have found that at times when it wouldn't be appropriate to share my thoughts – such as in the middle of the night or in class or when sharing would cross a boundary – even if I am very excited about my thoughts and *want to share them this instant*, writing them down in a small pocket-sized book helps ease my mind. That way the thoughts will not be forgotten, and I can always share them later in an appropriate way, in an appropriate context. My smaller book helped me develop important self-containment skills.

 ## Korrie

Korrie finds art to be very helpful in her recovery. She routinely uses it as a distraction, doing art projects instead of using her symptoms, especially after meals. She put together a "grounding box" which has become her first line of defense against her eating disorder.

"I have a box of things for when my symptoms are really bad, and when I'm struggling, I'll pull something out to help me," she says. The box is full of CDs, favorite movies, books, affirmations, a journal and candles. Recently Korrie began a scrapbook which she also keeps in her grounding box. "It takes my mind out of my symptoms and then I'm able to be mindful in something else."

One Saturday night Korrie was excited to go out with her friends. They had an exciting evening planned. But then Korrie got a text message saying that the plans were canceled. She was devastated.

"I got really upset," Korrie recalls, describing the self-destructive urges that rapidly bubbled to the surface. "I went to the box and used the scrapbook. I opened it and started coloring it. It was a much better choice than acting on my symptoms."

Art

Sometimes it can be difficult to put struggles into words. Using art may help you clarify what you are feeling, what you are thinking, and what work remains to be done.

℘ Jessica

After learning from her nutritionist that her weight had gone up a bit too quickly, Jessica was devastated. (For the complete story see Chapter 5.) Frantically, she searched for her friend Aimee. Aimee would know how to make this right. Although at first she could not find her friend, Aimee eventually found Jessica. The two of them talked as they walked to art therapy. They took the long way.

Once at art therapy, Jessica and Aimee met up with Dianne, the third member of their "dynamic trio." The three of them spent a lot of time together, virtually inseparable, and were instrumental parts of each other's recovery. The art therapist saw that Jessica was distressed and handed her a block of thick modeling clay to help her get out her frustration.

Jessica took the clay and pounded it, kneaded it, twisted it. Then she made a person out of it. The person was intended to be a clay version of Jessica herself. There were six layers from head to toe. Jessica painted each layer a different color to express how she felt about those body parts, much the way she had done previously with her therapist. When she was finished she wrote down all the things she hated about that body part and why she chose its color.

Still upset, but somewhat calmer, Jessica wrote a letter to her nutritionist expressing her hurt and concern that she had let Jessica's weight "climb too high too soon." Together they were able to put it into perspective and work through the challenge.

Art is a powerful form of expression that can give voice to your thoughts and feelings in a way that words cannot. This mode of creative expression can also be used at all stages of life and recovery for self-exploration, decision making, and as a visual reminder of various points along your life journey.

Aurora

After a stressful move Aurora was struggling immensely. She saw her therapist but continued to struggle. She had begun to slip badly and was stuck in a place of ambivalence. Did she want to continue down this road of self-destruction or did she want to fight to regain her health and strength? She honestly didn't always know. She knew she had to get out of the state of anguish she was in, but she also knew that she had not been making that choice nor taking any steps towards developing a better life.

Then, after a particularly difficult night filled with pain and self-loathing, an idea popped into Aurora's mind to create a collage. She hadn't used art to express herself in a very long time but she was drawn to the power of this collage...

Aurora created two worlds – one of desolation and despair and one of laughter and light. The lower world was dreary and barren, uninviting. It was filled to the brim with frustration and hate. A silhouette of a woman could be seen in this world. A dark representation of Aurora's current state.

But there was hope...

The upper world consisted of vibrant color and love. A white horse stood amongst the beautiful colors and inspiring quotes, a look of determination in its eyes. Aurora believes that horses, especially white horses, are spiritual creatures. She believes they are sensitive and can feel emotions – both hers and their own. When Aurora rides horses she connects with them on a spiritual level.

The horse in Aurora's collage knew where it was going and it wasn't going to stop. It was strong and steady and going to achieve its dreams. This was the world Aurora was struggling to enter.

She could make the move at any time. Although a line separated the two worlds, it was not so much a barrier as it was a reminder of a choice. The line consisted of a simple phrase which succinctly summed up her dilemma: "You must choose."

The collage served as a visual representation of the choices that lay before Aurora and her ability to make those choices. Tapping into your talents, be it art or music or dance or anything else, helps you along your individual path of recovery. It guides you away from identifying with your eating disorder. It reinforces your self-concept in a healthy way and, in a sense, reintroduces you to yourself.

Movement

So much of the struggle of an eating disorder is focused on the body. Therapeutic dance and movement gives voice to the body as the movement itself becomes a symbolic representation of behavioral and thought patterns. Movement therapy helps people work *with*, rather than *against*, their natural patterns.

According to dance movement therapist Susan Kleinman, it's not about what actions you take, but rather *how* you take those actions. Movement therapy is about thinking like a detective rather than as a patient. It helps you explore cognitively what's going on experientially. If you are not sure what's bothering you or where to begin a healing process, it gives you a place to start and a structure to follow. As you move, you collect clues to discover what's going on. You explore and acknowledge the truth even if you have no explanation for that truth. "Whys" take away from feeling. Acknowledgement is the acceptance of discovery. Discovery is always authentic in that it comes from *you*. As you integrate your discoveries and acknowledge the connection between your actions in movement therapy and familiar patterns and events in your life, a transformation takes place inside of you.

Dance movement therapy is about unfolding in an organic way. Movements are more than simple black and white actions. They are ways to communicate messages. During movement therapy we reflect our messages empathically. There is always communication present. We connect with others. When we recognize that we don't have to search outside ourselves for the answers, we can reflect inwardly.

Susan demonstrated this to me through the creation of two new movement exercises. We stood facing a chair in an otherwise empty room.

"Approach the chair," Susan said to me.

"What?" I asked.

"Approach the chair," she repeated.

I looked at the chair. I felt silly. What was I supposed to do? I stared at the chair. I looked at it from different angles. I carefully formulated a plan in my mind before finally walking briskly up to the chair and sitting down.

Susan asked me, "What did you just do? What was the process?"

"I wanted to figure out what to do before I did it," I told her.

"Hmm…" she said thoughtfully, "Where else in your life have you thought about what to do before acting?"

I thought for a moment and told her that it's a familiar pattern in my life. I'm a planner. I like to consider my options carefully before choosing a course of action. I acted similarly many times in the past in situations ranging from making plans for Saturday night to choosing a graduate school program. I think things through but once I have a plan I jump right into it.

"What can you do to work with your natural pattern?" Susan asked.

"I can make sure I have enough time to consider my options and mentally prepare my decisions," I answered.

This five-minute exercise touched on my decision-making process but it can be used in many different ways.

For another movement activity you will need a large yoga ball – the kind you can sit on. Place the ball in the middle of the room, making sure there is plenty of space around it in all directions. Sit on the ball for a few moments. Take an action on the ball – try a few. Ask yourself the following questions:

- How do you approach the ball?

- What do you notice happens when you sit on the ball?

- What do you experience in your body?

- What actions do you take on the ball?

- What did you discover? Why is it important?

- Explore your relationship with the ball: What does it represent? What does the floor represent? The air around you?

Finding a combination of creative means – art, music, and writing – that helps you cope is worthwhile in that it aids your progression in more stable times, and it also helps keep you from sliding back into old negative patterns during shaky times. You may even find it beneficial to put together a collection of creative and soothing items in one place and keep it nearby.

Door to Recovery

This exercise was created by psychologist Dr. Jennifer Nardozzi and dance movement therapist Susan Kleinman. They created the exercise to be used during one of Renfrew's "Rewriting Our Stories" events. Participants formed small groups and discussed a metaphoric door to recovery. We began by comparing barriers to recovery to a locked door. Questions for discussion included:

- What door remains locked in your recovery?

- What does the door to your recovery look like?

- What is the key to unlocking the door?

- What keeps you from opening the door?

- What lies beyond the door?

An art project followed in which participants were given journals and told to draw the door on the first page. On the following pages they were to write and draw all the things that lay waiting for them once they opened the door. As the day went on they could add to the list of positive things waiting for them on the other side.

I led one of the first discussion groups using this format. A common concern among group members was that many did not know what lay beyond their doors to recovery. They had been struggling with their eating disorders for many years and feared the unknown of a life without it. They told me the eating disorder was the only life they knew and they couldn't even imagine giving it up. I told them that they didn't need to know exactly what their lives in recovery would be like but I asked the group to think of a concrete scene – a snapshot – of recovery. One woman said that to her a moment in recovery would include petting her cat and watching television without worrying about food or body image.

This struck a chord in the other members of the group and they began coming up with their own snapshots of recovery.

In the midst of an eating disorder recovery can seem daunting. People with eating disorders often wonder how it is possible to go an entire day, hour, or even minute without thinking about food or body image or numbers. When the eating disorder has become the only life you know – when it has become your identity – it makes sense that imagining a life beyond the door to recovery is challenging. Don't worry if you can't pinpoint everything you want your life to be. Simply begin with a snapshot – one scene of recovery…

Chapter 8

CONNECTING SPIRITUALLY

"Listen from the inside out."

– Dr. Jennifer Nardozzi

When facing challenges and struggles in life, many people turn to their faith to help them succeed. The way I like to think of it is that on my own I can *push* through a struggle, but when I draw on my faith and spirituality I can *pull* through. *Pushing* means I am utilizing only my own strength and exerting my own energy to push away from a struggle. *Pulling*, by contrast, means that even in the midst of a challenge I am already connecting to something on the other side – something greater and stronger – and in doing so I am drawing on that power as I *pull* myself through the struggle toward something better.

Spirituality means many things to many people. Some draw strength from their religious faith, others find serenity in nature, and still others appreciate the value of connection – with a higher power, with others, and with themselves. For many people spirituality is a journey through life itself, complete with its own sets of ups and downs – periods of longing and yearning, and periods of peace and inspiration.

My spirituality is strongly linked to my religious faith. Being brought up in an Orthodox Jewish family means that religion and spirituality have played a central role in my life from the time I was born. My family's commitment to our faith in God and to the traditions set forth by our ancestors influence every decision we make – from what food we eat to the ways in which we handle emergencies.

My childhood is full of warm memories relating to Judaism – lighting Hanukkah candles with my family beside a mountain of wrapped presents atop our piano, studying for my bat mitzvah, and enjoying the most pleasant and fun Passover Seders I have ever known. As a child and pre-teen I loved my Judaic studies courses at school and even voluntarily attended classes after-hours as part of my school's extra-curricular learning program. Having been raised in accordance with my family's faith, I had my spirituality spoon-fed to me as a child. As a teenager I longed to "be my own person" and "find my own way." That was when I began to question my faith and where I belonged.

After high school I traveled to Israel, as is common in Orthodox Jewish circles, with the intention of exploring and discovering my own relationship with, and place in, the Orthodox Jewish world. I spent a year and a half abroad. I learned a lot and I grew in my religious observance. I developed a greater appreciation for the culture and history behind my faith.

When I came home from my study abroad program in Israel in the midst of a relapse, one of my – and my family's – key concerns about my treatment was how I would be able to maintain an Orthodox Jewish life. Would there be kosher food? Would I be able to observe the Sabbath and holidays? We consulted our rabbi who advised me that I needed to follow my doctors' orders – even if they seemed to contradict my faith – as my eating disorder was a matter of life or death. In Judaism saving a life takes precedence over all other commandments.

Luckily, I found a treatment center that was not only a terrific match for my physical, mental, and emotional needs, but for my religious and spiritual needs as well. At Renfrew all of my meals were brought in from a kosher restaurant and then portioned out to meet my specific meal plan requirements. Renfrew was sensitive to my religious observance and accommodated me during every step of my treatment. My rabbi walked me through the religious aspects of treatment and helped me stay connected to my community and lifestyle even while I spent time physically removed from it.

Although on the surface I appeared to be strong in my faith and commitment, I was struggling inside. Sometime toward the middle of my stay at Renfrew I had my first meeting with an aftercare counselor whose job it was to help me arrange an adequate aftercare plan for when I would leave Renfrew. During that introductory meeting I was asked what I wanted my life to look like after I left treatment.

Up until that point I'd been planning to continue working toward my bachelor's degree in psychology and then go on to graduate school for a doctoral degree in clinical psychology. It was a plan I'd developed at the end of high school and even though I was no longer sure of my desire to become a clinical psychologist, I felt that in my second year of college I'd already "come too far" to turn back.

When the aftercare counselor asked me to reconsider my goals and dreams, I told her "I don't know what I want to do in college." And then, while I was at it, "I don't even know if I want to go back to school…" I started questioning everything about my life. If I could change one thing, why not change *everything*? Rambling on and on about the changes I possibly wanted to make, I suddenly fell quiet as I hit a blaring red-light in my mind – *what if I want to change my religious lifestyle?*

Later that evening as I mentally reviewed the aftercare meeting, I was struck by a sudden wave of terror – *what if I don't believe in God?* I wondered. *What if I'm alone in this world and no one is watching over me?* And then, even scarier, *how can I face my family and my community if I no longer believe?*

For the most part I pushed the thoughts out of my mind. They were too scary and painful to entertain. Yet they remained in the back of my mind long after my time at Renfrew. For a long time I simply went through the motions of a religious life without any passion behind it. There was the added complication of having relapsed in the midst of religious growth and having to deal with the negative associations that entailed. Sadly, I contented myself with following the rules, often without a proper understanding, and keeping my doubts and questions mostly to myself. During this time I had *religion* but not *spirituality*.

I tried to regain my pre-eating disorder enthusiasm for Judaism but I knew I couldn't do it alone. Every so often I met with my rabbi to discuss my religious growth and where I wanted to be spiritually. It seemed as though I was getting nowhere and I grew extremely frustrated with my perceived lack of progress. Then one summer night I heard a Hebrew song that I hadn't heard since my first year in Israel, years before. I heard the song for the first time as a high school student on a Jewish youth program. I loved it then and felt it held some sort of power for me. When I arrived in Israel I met a girl who had the song on her iPod. We listened to it over and over again one night in the dorms. After leaving Israel during my relapse I didn't listen to the song for years. Shortly after my college graduation I lay awake in bed into the wee hours, longing for spiritual inspiration. I remembered the song from years back and downloaded it onto my own iPod. As I listened to the song for the first time in nearly five years, I was overcome with emotion. A few seconds into the opening melody I thought to myself, "This song was written to bring me back…"

I felt inspired and connected with all of my years of searching. There was hope and light and the feeling was indescribably powerful. At that moment I found the beauty in Judaism again and I knew I was not holding the status quo for my family. My faith and spirituality are something I treasure. They are rooted deep within me.

This flash of inspiration may appear to have come about on its own, but I firmly believe that it was a result of my honest effort and searching. I believe that when I try my hardest and manage those things which are within my realm of influence, the right doors will open at the right times. It may not always happen in the way that I expect, and it may not be predictable or even logical, but I believe it will happen. In my experience it always has, just as it did in this case. After two years of searching for inspiration, I never expected the inspiration to come through a song at 4:00 am, but that's the way it happened.

One thing I knew for certain was that a flash of inspiration like I experienced does not last long and it was up to me to make something of it. Inspiration is all too often a fleeting phenomenon unless immediate action is taken. In my case I used the inspiration I felt after hearing the song as a springboard of rediscovery. I began attending Judaic studies classes for adults in my community and learning Torah with a friend over the phone.

About a year later I drew on my new understanding of inspiration. In the midst of possibly my toughest struggle against my eating disorder in over three years, I had a flash of inspiration and wrote myself a letter from my "healthy voice" (see Chapter 4). I knew the clarity and inspiration would soon fade and that the letter had to be written right there and then. And so, during my most intense graduate course of the semester, psychopathology, I took the time to spell out my thoughts and really detail the reasons why I had to stay strong in my recovery. I knew exactly what I needed to hear and I also knew that no one would read my mind and say it to me, so I said it to myself. And what do you know? It was exactly what I needed to hear!

When you feel inspired, know that the inspiration itself presents you with choices: Will you simply have an inspired moment? Or will you *use* your inspiration to catapult yourself to greatness? If you choose the latter option, decide on a simple, definitive action to concretize your experience. If you are inspired to achieve a greater degree of recovery, or a more fulfilling social life or any other aspiration, think of one way you can achieve your goal. Maybe you will stay away from body-checking behaviors. Maybe you will challenge yourself to go out with friends instead of isolating yourself. Whatever your ultimate objective, set a simple, manageable goal. You may even find that the confidence arising from the achievement of your goal provides you with additional inspiration!

 ## Aurora

During residential treatment for her eating disorder at the age of twenty, Aurora received the heartbreaking news that her father passed away. During a moment of intense pain, her therapist handed her a stuffed bear in an attempt to comfort her.

"This is a Reiki Bear," her therapist explained, "It is infused with the spiritual healing power of Reiki. I want you to hold on to it for as long as you need it."

Aurora took the bear, although she did not understand the meaning of Reiki. Raised in a Catholic home, Aurora knew about going to church and confession, although those things never rang true for her. It took her until her teenage years – after the tragic loss of her brother and her family's dispersal – to connect with her own form of spirituality. Aurora's spirituality was a fluid concept. It changed and evolved with her as she grew older. She can now recall that her most intense moments of struggling were those very moments in which she lost touch with her spirituality. Likewise, her most intense moments of achievement and creativity were the moments in which she was the most in tune with her spirituality. At the moment her therapist handed her the Reiki bear, Aurora gratefully accepted. Upon hearing the news of her father's passing, Aurora was not spiritually connected. In fact she was spiritually *disconnected* during the entire span of her relapse leading to her admission to treatment. But somewhere, deep in her soul, Aurora yearned for a spiritual reawakening.

Years passed and Aurora still held the Reiki Bear in her possession. She felt bad as she had never intended to keep the bear for this long. Then one day Aurora attended a Rewriting Our Stories event at the Renfrew Center where she had been treated and she decided to return the bear to her therapist. She brought the Reiki Bear, intending to give it back, but when she handed the bear over, her therapist told her to keep it.

"No," said Aurora, "You told me to keep the bear until I was ready to give it back. I'm ready." Aurora and her therapist stood in deep conversation for several minutes. Between the two of them they decided what to do with the Reiki Bear and a new tradition was born at Renfrew: Each week in the patient-run spirituality group, the Reiki Bear would be passed along to another patient who needed a little extra support and healing power. Aurora began the tradition by ceremoniously handing over the bear to a struggling patient in the room.

That same day, Aurora met a woman who was well-versed in Reiki. Several months later she attended her first Reiki circle. Knowing very little about Reiki, Aurora did not know what to expect as she sat down and closed her eyes in meditation. She had had a dream about her father the night before. It was a sad dream. She woke up crying and felt deeply saddened. Now in the Reiki circle, tears began streaming down her cheeks once more. Just as she raised a hand to her face to wipe away her tears, a Reiki healer came to her and began practicing Reiki on her. Aurora felt the healer place a crown on her head. It felt as though the crown was made of leaves. She thought of her father and it was as though their spirits connected.

The healer came to Aurora twice more throughout the meditation and each time Aurora felt the crown on her head. She felt better, she felt free. She began to tell herself positive things:

"I am connecting with my inner goddess."

"My light shines so bright."

"I have so much to share with the world."

Aurora felt incredible. After the Reiki circle ended she asked her friend about the crown the healer put on her head during meditation.

"What?" her friend asked her.

"The crown," Aurora pressed, "What is the significance of the crown they put on my head?"

Her friend stared at her incredulously. "The healers just use their hands," she explained, "There was no crown…" Then a look of amazement shone in her eyes.

Slowly, Aurora's friend explained to her the concept of the "crown chakra." Aurora later researched the Reiki chakras and learned that each one corresponded to a different part of the body. The crown chakra corresponded to the head and mind and meant complete connection to the universe as well as acknowledgement and acceptance of one's spirituality.

Aurora was blown away – she had really felt a crown of leaves on her head! In that moment Aurora knew this was no coincidence. She truly believed things were in divine order.

She decided to learn Reiki and become a Reiki master. The place where she attended the Reiki circle was holding a beginning Reiki workshop on the anniversary of her father's death – the day on which she first received the Reiki Bear. Aurora found great meaning in the timing and knew that it was meant to be. Her feelings inside were phenomenal and unexplainable. Her inspiration was strong. It was a powerful feeling – a feeling of power!

"Trust the universe." This simple phrase contains the wisdom that Dr. Jennifer Nardozzi often shares with her patients. "Things really are in divine order," she explains. There is a meaning and a purpose to our lives even if – in the moment – nothing seems to make any sense. Dr. Nardozzi encourages clients to look for the deeper meaning in their struggles. "There must be a higher purpose for going through all of this," she asserts. The challenge is finding it. There is no single right answer. If an answer, or several answers, ring true for you and inspire you towards continued progress, accept them and keep moving onward. Use the meaning in your struggles to help you face challenges and fears, and as a catalyst for growth.

Dr. Nardozzi subscribes to the belief of Anita Johnson, author of *Eating in the Light of the Moon*, that an eating disorder is a messenger of the soul. This powerful concept has helped many individuals not only conquer their symptoms, but also learn to use to their benefit the very demons that haunt them. In this way, a negative experience is transformed into a source of self-knowledge and understanding – a source of power.

"When a person has an eating disorder," states Dr. Nardozzi, "it is a signal that something is off-center spiritually. If we can meet our spiritual needs, there is no longer a need for the eating disorder. Our spiritual needs are akin to a void within us." Dr. Nardozzi cautions that the void must be used properly. Don't fill the gap with just anything (i.e. symptoms). Instead, search for what it is you truly lack; learn the lessons your soul is trying to teach you; discover your true needs and meet them in a deep and real way. Play an active role in your recovery and in your life.

The juxtaposition of my story and Aurora's story reveals an interesting discovery: While my spirituality is rooted in ancient Jewish tradition and hers is rooted in connection with her inner self, with others, and with the universe, our stories actually run quite parallel to each other's – our childhood experience of having our spirituality spoon-fed to us, our teenage searching for our own place, the disconnection we experienced during times of intense struggling, and finally, the rediscovery of a spiritual life in recovery.

Andrew

Andrew made a pact. He would go into treatment one last time. If that didn't work he would kill himself. Treatment worked this time but it was no coincidence.

"I didn't need to kill myself," says Andrew. "What helped me all along was my faith that there had to be a reason for it. It's not for me to give up. God has a plan for me. I didn't think it was a very fair plan, but it wasn't for me to take my own life."

Andrew used to go to church regularly. He found great peace in the church. It was a sanctuary for Andrew. He regularly prayed for the strength to continue towards his recovery.

"I prayed everyday for recovery and eventually I got there" says Andrew. "I still pray."

Some people can easily identify their spiritual sides. Others find this more challenging. When asked about her spirituality, for example, Korrie initially replied, "I'm not exactly a 'spiritual' person." When asked to give the matter a bit more thought, Korrie realized that despite her self-proclaimed non-spiritual nature, there were some spiritually-infused concepts with which she could relate. Reflecting on Dr. Nardozzi's statement that an eating disorder is a form of spiritual hunger, Korrie found that this idea deeply resonated with her. Throughout her eating disorder, Korrie was hungry for acceptance and love from others as well as from herself. Korrie also believes that there is meaning and purpose within her struggles.

Korrie

At a frat house party with her friends, Korrie found herself miserable. Cute guys were flirting with her friends but ignoring her. While her friends had the time of their lives, Korrie stood in the corner of the room dejected, her arms crossed and an angry, hurt expression on her face. She was not enjoying the party one bit.

Korrie's first reaction was to tell herself that the boys had obviously ignored her because she was ugly and fat. In order to gain their approval she would have to diet and exercise and lose weight. Then she would be attractive and people would like her. Before these distorted thoughts turned into symptoms, Korrie caught herself and realized that her current train of thought was not a healthy one.

Working with her therapist, she came to understand that the real reason behind her perceived rejection by others at the party stemmed from the way in which she had presented herself that night. Who wants to approach someone who is all upset? People go to parties in order to have a good time. No one wants to be bogged down by another person's misery at a party. People like to be with happy people!

Put in this way, Korrie was able to step back and see that there was no personal affront in the others' behavior. It wasn't that her friends were better than her or smarter than her or more attractive than her. It was simply that Korrie gave off vibes that said, "Don't mess with me." Maybe other people were just giving her the space they thought she needed. Maybe they didn't want to expend the energy it would take to try to cheer her up. In any case, this was a matter completely within Korrie's power to influence.

Knowing what choices you have and what outcomes are within your realm of influence is crucial. Korrie could have continued to blame her unhappiness on others but instead she fought to take charge. She worked with her therapist to develop more effective interpersonal skills and now she enjoys a much happier and more fulfilling social life. Realizations like Korrie's – that she was largely the source of her own unhappiness – can be difficult to accept but can lead the way to positive change. Inspiration does not only come from pleasant events and insights. Sometimes adverse situations lead to increased awareness and motivation. Sometimes inspiration comes from places you least expect…

The Renfrew Center of Florida has an outdoor sanctuary called the Healing Garden. It's a quiet garden with plants and rocks, a swing and hammock, artwork, a fountain, and several other soothing elements. It is known as a safe haven by patients and staff alike and is used for peaceful relaxation and unwinding as well as for creativity and inspiration.

Where did the idea for the Healing Garden come from?

"At one point," says Dr. Nardozzi, "there was no Healing Garden, just a grassy knoll. The idea to create the garden developed out of staff meetings which aimed to promote spiritual healing. Someone had the thought to ask former patients what would be helpful to have in the garden, so at the next alumnae reunion they passed a rock around a circle and each former patient said something they wanted from the garden:

"A sacred place."

"A place where people can connect in any way they choose."

"A place to give people a break from the business of treatment."

"What actually emerged was amazing," says Dr. Nardozzi. "It was like energy was drawn to the space. Clients met there with their families. Then people started spontaneously donating to the garden – a fountain, gazebo, plants, a hammock. People wanted to give back to the garden that had given them something during their treatment."

The Healing Garden project took on a life of its own. Garden rituals were put in place to honor the beginning and end of treatment. The two ceremonies were linked by small rocks that provided continuity and connection between the beginning and the end. Each patient chose a rock out of a basket upon arrival. The rock would have a special word painted on it and the patient would articulate what meaning it held for her.

The Healing Garden rocks became a sacred tradition at Renfrew. What's interesting though, is that this trend didn't stop with the patients. Dr. Nardozzi and other Renfrew professionals take Healing Garden rocks with them to conferences around the world.

"It never fails," says Dr. Nardozzi, "Professionals love this ritual!"

During one particularly eventful conference, the rocks took on a new meaning, inspiring the professionals in attendance. Dr. Nardozzi, dance movement therapist Susan Kleinman, and a Renfrew alumna arrived at the conference with over three hundred Healing Garden rocks ready for the closing ceremony. Somehow, though, the rocks had gotten lost in transit. The whole ritual was based on the rocks so they decided they must track them down! By the time the rocks were located, they had been through a lot and the painted-on words had rubbed off and faded. The Renfrew staff members spent hours well into the night repainting the three hundred rocks before the following day's ceremony.

As frustrating as it was to have to repaint the words, a certain amount of meaning was gleaned through the experience. Dr. Nardozzi's group compared the rocks to the clients they see: When they arrive for treatment their identities are worn and faded. It is the therapists' job to help them find themselves again. Upon hearing this story years later, one former patient added a twist to the story – when the words on the rocks faded they were still *there*, just harder to read. So too, the clients do not *lose* their identities, rather they must find and *clarify* them.

How many times do people go into treatment expecting to emerge as a "whole new person?" It doesn't work that way nor should it. You are you. You are already who you are supposed to be. Healthy self-improvement should not be confused with attempts to change who you are.

And to think that all of this insight and inspiration was gained from a frustrating night of painting rocks! There are other points of spiritual interest in this story as well, specifically symbolism and giving back.

Symbolism is a common theme in treatment. During my treatment I made a containment box, chose rocks out of a basket, and made a "sculpture" of my family life by carefully positioning fellow patients in residential treatment. The family sculpture actually is a human sculpture in which fellow patients assume various positions and distances from each other in order to portray a specific family's dynamics. Sometimes symbolism means taking something concrete and using it to learn about something deeper, sometimes it means using an everyday object as a springboard for more advanced thought, and sometimes it means having something to hold onto to remind you of your motivation and will to thrive.

Jessica

> Jessica's residential therapist gave her a little book of uplifting and encouraging quotes. The book, called *Believe in Yourself*, by Beth Mende Conry, is bright and colorful. The cover is full of flowers and attached is a yellow ribbon with a flower at the end that is intended as a bookmark. Jessica's therapist had bookmarked a specific page that read, "And the day came when the risk to remain tight in a bud was more painful than the risk it took to blossom."
>
> Flowers became Jessica's symbol of recovery and the quote became her mantra. Now whenever Jessica sees a blossoming flower – even if it is only a picture – she feels the beauty and power of her recovery.

For me the Healing Garden rocks from Renfrew hold great power. They are not so valuable in and of themselves, but when they are invested with a person's thoughts, feelings, and energy they take on a whole new level of importance.

I personally have five Healing Garden rocks in my possession. Each one holds special meaning to me because of the time when it was received and what I was going through. In *One Life* I discuss my experience with my first rock, "Try," which was given to me at the beginning of my residential treatment.

Two years later I received my second rock. It was the morning of my interview day for admission to my top choice graduate school and I was understandably nervous. I gave a short presentation at the Renfrew Center that morning and afterwards I was invited to choose a rock as an honorary member of the group. My rock said "Hope." My interpretation was that after *trying* my hardest and doing all that is in my control, sometimes I have to let go a little bit and *hope* for the best. (I got in and now attend the school!)

I got my third and fourth rocks on the same day at the annual Renfrew reunion. One said "See" and the other said "Mitzvah." "See" taught me to open my eyes and experience what is really there and to shed my preconceived notions and cognitive distortions about what *should* be or what *will* happen. "See" helped me take a step back and notice the positives in my life, especially those for which I had worked hard. If you're ever buffed a wood floor you know that you can't see the progress you are making until you literally take a few steps back and view the contrast between the buffed parts and the not-yet-buffed parts of the floor. It's the same with changes in life. Most real-life changes occur gradually in subtle stages. Often it takes looking back over a long period of time and viewing the contrast between where you were and where you are now in order to see how far you've come.

"Mitzvah" is the Hebrew word meaning "commandment" and is often used to mean "good deed," especially in a religious sense. It held meaning to me as I received this rock during my spiritual awakening. I took it as a point of transition – I was moving toward a full life and reintegrating lost elements. It was also significant as a reminder of the connection between seemingly separate parts of my life. I never expected to see the word "Mitzvah" on a Healing Garden rock, yet there it was! My religious life and my recovery life were not so separate after all. There was a sense of unity as I turned the rock over in my hands.

My fifth rock says "Whole." I picked it out of a small lace bag at another Renfrew event. By this point I'd been living on my own in Florida for several weeks attending graduate school. I had a full social life and had successfully reconnected to my spiritual side. It represented to me the need to live a full life, with attention paid to all parts – social, spiritual, physical, emotional…

In each of the five rocks I found a message. Like many therapy tools, the rocks served to help me access the wisdom within me. It was already there, the rocks simply brought it to the surface. Perhaps the most important "rock" I have is not a Healing Garden rock at all and it has no words on it. It is a small shell I found on the beach while celebrating my twenty-first birthday with my friend Danielle. The shell is shaped like a ball and there is something inside of it that moves around when you shake it. I originally wanted to crack it open and see what was inside, but in talking to Danielle I decided to leave it whole. The shell came to symbolize the mysteries of life. Curiosity is a good thing but it's also okay not to know or understand everything. The shell also demonstrates my growing independence and self-determination. No one handed it to me and no one told me what it meant. No one even suggested that it *had* a special meaning. I chose it for myself. Of all the "rocks" in my collection, the shell is the only one I carry with me in my purse wherever I go. I think that's because to me it represents real life, with real friends, and real dreams.

 ## Lexi

Even as a little girl Lexi dreamed of saving the world. She reflects that her desire for "world peace" was echoed by many characters in the movie *Miss Congeniality*. She wanted to attack the "big picture," solving massive crises and making a big, noticeable difference. Unfortunately, in always considering the "big picture" Lexi often felt small and insignificant. She hid behind other people's problems because, to Lexi, other people's problems seemed bigger than her own. How could she struggle with her "puny little challenges" when others' challenges were so much greater?

Despite her belief that her problems were insignificant, Lexi often found herself miserable and angry at God. One night as she lay awake in bed filled with negativity and eating disorder thoughts, tears flowing down her face, Lexi turned to God and said aloud, "Why are you putting me through all of this? It's painful. It's hard. What is the purpose? What is *my* purpose?" It was then that Lexi intuitively understood a great truth: The purpose of her struggles – and the purpose of her life – could not be seen through the lens of her eating disorder. While this frustrated Lexi immensely, she knew that she needed to get well before there could be true understanding.

Her journey of faith eventually led her on an ever-winding path towards finding herself and her life's purpose. Lexi likens the experience to that of a roller-coaster ride, but admits that as she approached new levels of recovery and her symptoms decreased, God seemed to open more and more doors for her. What began as a simple opportunity to help out with her church's youth program evolved into a calling to help younger churchgoers and to show them unconditional love and acceptance. When she moved away for graduate school she made sure to find another church where she could lead youth groups.

Moving away, starting graduate school, and working with a new group of teenagers in a new town was a huge transition for Lexi who spent the majority of her life in one place. Stepping outside her comfort zone, Lexi reminded herself that she had made it through tougher times and she could surely handle this transition as well. In retrospect she could see that her challenges hadn't been so puny and little after all, but rather than drown her in despair, this recognition inspired hope for the future – she made it through in the past and she could make it through now. She was inspired also by the fact that "little ol' Lexi" was making a "big ol' difference" in helping to create a ministry that was changing teenagers' lives right before her eyes. She knew that what was having the biggest impact on her group was the personal connection she established with each of them. Furthermore, she knew that the reason she was able to do this work in the first place was because of her commitment to get well and stay well. This success was merely a link in the chain of her recovery; her recovery was a link in the chain of her life; and her life was, in fact, part of the "big picture."

In finding her place – in a small rural town, going to school, and working with teenagers at her new church – Lexi discovered that she was exactly where she was supposed to be all along. The struggles, the feelings of inadequacy, the trials and triumphs – they each served as a motivator for Lexi to grow into her full potential. Each step in her journey had a purpose, and though she does not know the specific purpose of every step, Lexi has learned to trust the process and to know that as long as she tries her hardest, God will lead her wherever she is meant to be.

Saving the world starts with helping to heal one person.

And very often, that one person is you.

Chapter 9

COPING WITH TRAUMA AND LOSS

"You can't let go of something that
you don't acknowledge."

– Regina Lukens

The goal of recovery from trauma, in a sense, can be boiled down to learning from the past, bettering the future, and living in today. Many people suffering from eating disorders are also survivors of trauma. The connection between the two is somewhat complicated and different for every person; however, there is one common underlying factor: An eating disorder often serves as a form of pseudo-protection from trauma, which can result in powerful feelings of guilt, shame, anger, sadness, and disgust. When these feelings become overwhelming, an eating disorder can "help" a person cope by numbing his or her emotions.

Because of the tendency for people with eating disorders to numb their feelings through their food-related symptoms when attempting to cope with trauma, the issue of where to begin in therapy is a tricky one. While the underlying issues for many people involve traumatic events in their pasts, jumping straight into treatment to resolve past trauma can be counterproductive when a person's eating disorder symptoms are still rampant. In fact this can serve to exacerbate the problem.

"People use [eating disorder] symptoms because they work," says Regina Lukens, social worker and trauma specialist. Trauma work is triggering by nature. It involves learning to sit through extremely uncomfortable feelings. It sometimes happens that people are more motivated to work through their issues of trauma than their eating disorders. Regina cautions her clients that doing trauma work *will* intensify eating disorder urges. Regina also explains that trauma has many layers and they are all interconnected. While working on one layer, another layer can get triggered and then there is more that is accessible to work on. Discovering new layers of trauma work can also trigger eating disorder thoughts, presenting a formidable challenge. However, it need not place your recovery in jeopardy. If you begin to struggle with symptoms or get stuck it is crucial that you discuss this with your therapist. You may need to slow the pace of your trauma work, lessen the intensity, or approach it in a different way.

According to Regina a person must first be willing to stop using symptoms before there is the possibility of healing from trauma. "In order for there to be healing, there must first be safety," she says. Unless you are physically safe, you cannot begin the healing process. Not only must the trauma be over and in the past in order for the healing process to begin, but also the eating disorder symptoms must be at least somewhat in check. This does not mean that you have to be completely symptom-free, but it does mean that you must be maintaining at least some level of recovery.

Eating disorders keep people in survival mode, in much the same way as a trauma. In this sense, it is not just about whether or not the actual trauma is over. If you are still hurting yourself then there cannot be true healing. This applies not only to symptoms of eating disorders but also to symptoms of trauma. Nightmares and flashbacks as well as risky and self-harming behavior can serve to re-victimize a person who has experienced a trauma or other painful or difficult experience in his or her life.

It is not only painful but also futile to work on issues of past trauma while fully engaging in eating disorder symptoms. The eating disorder takes the edge off feelings. It cushions a person from feeling the emotions necessary in order to truly work through trauma. In this type of situation the trauma and eating disorder can become self-perpetuating problems. One key goal is to separate food and feelings – to make food just food and feelings just feelings.

So what is trauma? According to therapist and trauma specialist Heidi Salonia trauma is "any experience or event that has a negative or lasting effect on self or psyche." Heidi goes on to differentiate between big "T" traumas and little "t" traumas. Big "T" traumas include vehicle accidents, rape, physical abuse, and sudden death. Little "t" traumas include surgeries, humiliation, bullying, and losing a friendship. There are no clear-cut criteria determining which specific events constitute traumas and which do not. It is not about the event itself, but rather about your experience of the event and your experience following the event. As Heidi points out, if the experience caused long-term negative effects, it was a trauma and needs to be dealt with as such.

Physical responses to trauma include changes in appetite or sleep patterns, hyper-arousal, aches and pains, heart palpitations, and sweating. Emotional responses to trauma include fear, guilt, rage, irritability, intrusive thoughts, night terrors, feelings of helplessness, and difficulty concentrating. Specific symptoms of trauma – such as flashbacks and dissociation – vary from person to person but according to Heidi they are almost always triggered by one of the five senses: sight, sound, touch, taste, and smell. If, for example, you suffered a medical trauma, the sight of medical equipment, the sound of a heart monitor, the taste of medication, the feeling of nausea, or the smell of a hospital may trigger trauma responses.

Dissociation causes a break in the connection between one's identity and one's thoughts and memories. Some dissociation is healthy and normal. "Dissociation is a coping mechanism we all have as humans," says Regina. Examples of mild dissociation include daydreaming and going on autopilot during a routine drive to work such that you do not recall much of the drive. Dissociation becomes a problem when it interferes with a person's ability to live a healthy, functional life. People subconsciously use dissociation to disconnect from feelings that are too painful, overwhelming, or unsafe to let themselves feel. While dissociation is a built-in human defense against life-threatening danger, it can misfire and occur during stable times long after a trauma has passed, becoming more of a danger in itself than a protection.

I once heard a story that poignantly illustrates this idea. The story was about a little girl who lived in a big house. A major storm was coming so the girl hid in the very center of the house, sheltered and safe. No windows – no openings at all. The storm ravaged the yard and even the outer parts of the house, but not that little room deep inside where the girl was hiding. In her little room she was safe. But when the storm passed and it was safe to go outside again, the little girl remained hidden in her room. She didn't dare venture out. She remained in the center room of the house, locked away by fear.

This fictional story is analogous to a trauma response in which survival instincts misfire.

Says Regina, "If you say in a fog too long you get lost." If you go through life in a fog, just going through the motions, disconnected, you can wind up in dangerous situations for lack of paying attention. You can also get yourself into emotional trouble by isolating.

In the case of trauma and eating disorders co-occurring, food can become a means of dissociation. The goal, says Regina, is to shift your relationship to how you feel emotionally. "When you're sad," she says, "don't go use food. Overwhelming grief doesn't mean you need to purge. You want to sit with the feelings, no matter how overwhelming they are." One way to ground yourself during such times is to place both feet on the floor. This gives you a sense of connection and security. Other means include playing with silly putty, squeezing a stress ball, and consciously noting things that you see, hear, smell, taste, and touch. Connect with your senses.

Flashbacks are periods during which a person re-lives a traumatic event. The recollection is so strong and so vivid that the person is unable to recognize that it is a memory and not the current reality. Flashbacks are usually triggered involuntarily and are accompanied by a rush of intense emotion – the same emotion experienced during the actual trauma. In effect, a flashback can actually re-traumatize a person. Contrary to a belief held by many, you do *not have to re-live trauma in order to heal*! The process of recovery is about emotional healing, and to do that you need not re-experience the pain.

A flashback is different from a memory. When you have a memory you know where you are. When you have a flashback you become so disoriented that you lose touch with the present moment and with your surroundings. Regina explains that "not all people who have been traumatized have flashbacks." And fortunately, "Flashbacks tend to be something you can learn not to have." Sometimes people purposely go into flashbacks in order to re-live it and experience the pain again. It keeps them "stuck" in the role of victim. This is particularly common in cases where there is a significant history of trauma. If this is a pattern that is familiar to you, then speak to your therapist. Know that there is no need to feel ashamed of it and there is help.

Nightmares are another common occurrence among survivors of trauma. They may be isolated or recurring dreams causing great distress, fear, and even panic. According to Regina, one way to manage nightmares and flashbacks is to rewrite the ending of the story. Of course, this is only meant for situations in which the trauma is *completely in the past.* (The trauma must be over. If it is not over, then your work is to seek appropriate help in ending it – such as getting out of an abusive relationship and achieving safety.) When you rewrite the ending of a nightmare or flashback, change it so that in the end you are not hurt nor in danger. You may also need to rewrite the *meaning* of the story in order to change the way you view it. For example, if you feel that a traumatic event like abuse was your fault then you can rework it in your mind to represent what you should have learned – or will learn – in therapy: Abuse is *never* your fault.

It is appropriate at this point to note that while what happened is not your *fault*, it *is* your *responsibility* to engage in the healing process.

Jessica

When Jessica was younger she experienced traumatic instances of verbal and physical abuse, both to herself and to others in her family. Like many others who have survived such ordeals, Jessica believed for a long time that she was somehow at fault for what happened and these faulty beliefs hurt her self-image and caused her to feel tremendous shame.

One such occurrence was a time when an abusive relative of Jessica's came after her in a drunken fit of rage, threatening to hurt her severely. Jessica's older brother came in between the two of them in order to protect Jessica and as a result he was the one who was hurt. The relative was eventually banned from the household and the abuse ceased.

For years Jessica carried around painful feelings of guilt and shame over what happened that day and on other occasions when her brother protected her in similar ways. She was afraid and ashamed to share her pain with others, including her mother and her therapist, because she believed it was her fault that her brother was regularly abused. Jessica also worried that even if she told her mother what happened, her mother may not believe her or she may confirm that it *was* Jessica's fault.

With the help of her therapist, Jessica finally shared what happened and began to learn the truth – that the abuse did not signify a problem with *Jessica*, but rather it signified a problem with her *relative*. When Jessica eventually unburdened herself of these horrific secrets she'd been keeping for years, she began to heal. Her mother helped her understand that the abuse was not her fault, nor was it specific to Jessica – this relative abused many members of the family, including Jessica's mother.

In time, Jessica internalized the positive, healthy messages of her mother and therapist and she learned to move past the trauma. It admittedly took a long time for Jessica to completely remove the belief that it was somehow her fault, but in time she unlearned those thought patterns and replaced them with new, healthier ones.

As is mentioned above, it can be very difficult to change the meaning of the story, or the ending of the story, in your mind. If the trauma, such as abuse, happened when you were young, or scared, or otherwise in a position of disadvantage or compromise, it can be a bit more challenging to redirect the ending. In such instances, Regina would advise you to bring someone else into the flashback – "Someone who possesses the ability to be strong in the face of whoever is hurting [you] and stop what is happening." Someone who can protect you. The protector can be a therapist, a friend, someone you just met, a superhero or other mythical embodiment of strength, a religious figure, or even an older or stronger version of yourself.

"Suggest this image in your mind before going to sleep in order to prevent nightmares," says Regina. "It can take some practice." The key is to use this method *before* a nightmare or flashback occurs. Get used to making the change in the story ahead of time. When you feel a flashback coming – and you can know when it's coming because of the physical symptoms, such as sweaty palms, a racing heart, and feeling not grounded – *that's* when you bring in your protector.

There are also more structured ways to manage these responses and even to prevent their occurrence. Both Heidi and Regina use certain practical exercises with their clients who have experienced trauma. Three exercises in particular – safe place, containment box, and spiral technique – can be practiced with or without a therapist. It is important to point out that all trauma-related exercises *must* be practiced during times when your stress levels are *low*. Once you can successfully de-escalate your stress from lower levels, you can begin to use these exercises when your stress level is higher. In other words, you need to build up to the point that you can use the exercises to deflect trauma responses.

Practical exercises
Safe place by Heidi Salonia
There are many variations of the safe place exercise, but one that is especially useful is the "Creating a Safe Place" exercise developed by Heidi Salonia over the course of several years, based on a number of sources. It is an eight-step, methodical guide to creating and using a safe place, and it can be used both when you

are calm and in times of stress. (This exercise belongs to therapist Heidi Salonia.)

1. *Image.* Identify an image of a safe place that you can easily bring up in your mind that creates a feeling of calmness and safety.

2. *Emotions and sensations.* Next, focus on the image, feel the emotions, and identify the location of the pleasing physical sensations in your body.

3. *Enhancement.* You may hum, rock, listen to music, nature, or use soothing tones to enhance the imagery and your emotions. Remember this is a place of safety and security for you.

4. *Experience.* Bring up the image of a place that feels safe and calm. Concentrate on where you feel the pleasant sensations in your body and allow yourself to enjoy them. Take a deep breath and focus on these sensations. "How do you feel now?"

5. *Cue word.* Identify a single word that fits the picture (e.g. "relax," "beach," "mountain," "trees") and rehearse this mentally while paying attention to the bodily sensations.

6. *Self-cuing.* Please complete the whole procedure on your own now, bringing up the image and the word and experiencing the positive feelings (both emotions and physical sensations). Use this procedure during times of stress.

7. *Cuing with disturbance.* Now bring up a minor annoyance that irritates you or makes you slightly uncomfortable. Notice the accompanying negative feelings. Repeat the

safe place exercise with your therapist until the negative feelings dissipate.

8. *Self-cuing with disturbance.* Bring up the disturbing thought once more and follow the safe place exercise but without the help of your therapist. Concentrate on your safe place until you feel relaxed.

Containment box by Regina Lukens

Regina Lukens uses the technique below with clients who are beginning to work on issues of trauma and advises them to go back to it during times of stress. She teaches clients that there are certain times when it is appropriate to deal with issues of trauma, such as in therapy, and certain times when it is inappropriate, such as at mealtimes. The goal of this exercise is to help clients "contain" their difficult and overwhelming thoughts and feelings and to put them somewhere safe where they can be retrieved later on.

1. Imagine a container, such as a file cabinet, lockbox, mp3 player, or a therapist's office. Your containment box should be something secure to which you can entrust difficult thoughts and feelings. Your container can be nearly anything, although Regina cautions clients never to use a coffin, as it defeats the purpose of the exercise. The idea is that you will come back to the contents of your container at a later time. A coffin signifies a certain finality and unwillingness to accept or own your thoughts, feelings, and experiences. "[Using a coffin as your container] invalidates your experience," says Regina. Many of your experiences of trauma may have been invalidated or denied at one point or another. Using a coffin perpetuates an inability to heal. Says Regina, "You can't let go of something that you don't acknowledge."

2. Choose a body part that feels uncomfortable and pair the discomfort with a color. Then prepare to metaphorically put it (the color) somewhere. "You don't actually have to know what 'it' is," says Regina. "The whole point of containment is to turn down the volume on overwhelming experiences… [and] later go back and take them out and face them." Regina has her clients sit with their feet placed firmly on the floor, as this serves as a sort of grounding experience in itself, and begin to imagine the color they selected coming out of their chosen body part like a stream of light. As you imagine the colored light exiting your body, direct it into your open container. If you have trouble visualizing the light leaving your body, or if it is not moving quickly enough, Regina recommends imagining a vacuum cleaner pulling it out of you and into your container.

3. When all of the color is in your containment box, close and lock your container. Then mentally put yourself in your safe place. With practice this exercise has helped many people manage feelings of discomfort and even ease their uncomfortable sensations.

Spiral technique by Heidi Salonia

This technique used by Heidi Salonia incorporates the work of Yosef Wolpe on subjective units of discomfort and uses a form of guided imagery in order to help people take charge of their stress levels. When thoughts and feelings are overwhelming, there can be a sense of hopelessness and helplessness – a feeling of being out of control. This exercise aims to help people take back their power by providing an alternate focus.

1. Close your eyes and make a mental note of how you feel in your body.

2. Bring to mind a slightly annoying or mildly disturbing thought and notice what you feel in your body and where you feel it. Don't do anything about it, don't respond to it – just notice it.

3. Imagine that this uncomfortable feeling is energy moving in a spiral. Notice in what direction the spiral is turning. Clockwise? Counterclockwise? Again, just notice.

4. Now, mentally move the spiral in the opposite direction and see what happens. Your stress level may have decreased and any negative sensation may have lessened or gone away.

Although these techniques were designed to help people cope with trauma responses, they can be used by anyone experiencing discomfort, disturbing thoughts, or anxiety. These exercises have proven useful in helping people stay grounded, ease their anxiety, and lower their stress levels.

Aside from these typical trauma responses there are long-term emotional effects that often accompany traumatic incidences. These may not cause the same kind of acute moments of danger, but are nonetheless important to address in therapy. For example, after losing a family member or friend there is a grief process that must take place. There is the added challenge of a significant loss creating a change in the family dynamics, in addition to having to cope with the grief of others. For example, if you were a child at the time of the loss, then you likely had to deal with grieving parents who were less present, emotionally, to care for you.

❦ Aurora

Aurora's family used to be a close, cohesive unit. They ate dinner together and were very involved in each other's lives. Then, when Aurora was fifteen years old, her brother suddenly died in a tragic car accident. The family was shattered.

They stopped eating dinner together. They stopped being a close-knit group and instead they dispersed, with each member of the family fending for themselves. A grieving fifteen-year-old, Aurora didn't know how to care for and nurture herself. The abrupt and drastic change in the family dynamics was a catalyst for the development of her unhealthy coping behaviors. Aurora's grieving parents had trouble caring for their surviving children. Aurora, unable to find the nurturance she so desperately needed from her family during such a difficult time, turned to drugs and eating disorder symptoms. She was also hurting herself physically. This was the first time Aurora lost anyone close to her and she did not have sufficient support. On a subconscious level she was trying to cope with all that she had lost – her brother, her close-knit family, her life as she knew it until that point. But at the time, Aurora had no idea why she suddenly had such trouble. She told herself she was flawed, horrible, a failure.

Four years after her brother's death, Aurora began to explore its impact on her and her family. She began to realize the profundity of it all and how it had been the starting point of her negative behaviors. Nonetheless she was not ready to work on the major issues when she entered residential treatment for the first time. It took her until her second time in treatment, when she lost her father to a serious illness, in order to begin to explore both losses.

At first Aurora was numb. Soon numbness gave way to bitterness and anger. She was furious with God. How could such terrible things happen to her family? They were so happy together – they didn't deserve to lose these two great men! Aurora cried. A lot. Although this was initially uncomfortable for her, she learned to come to terms with the crying and to let it be cleansing. She talked to her dad and her brother out loud. She listened to music that reminded her of her father. She tried to focus on the good memories and to write about them. She talked with her family about her father. She came to appreciate just how greatly her father and brother shaped who she was and how they still inspired her. Even though she lost them, she learned so much from them during the time that they were with her.

"I'm one really lucky person to have had them in my life for even a short time," says Aurora. "Some people don't have that at all… [I am] grateful to be blessed with those relationships. I will always have that with me."

Everyone deals with loss in their own way. Grief is a painful process that takes time. Like any process, it is not simply a direct movement towards peace. There are periods of tremendous anger and denial. There are times of questioning. Sometimes it hurts worse than other times. And hopefully, through the emotional twists and turns, there is acceptance.

Jessica

It was her senior year in high school and Jessica was in love. She had the most amazing boyfriend. His name was Rick. They had so much in common. Their personalities complemented each other's and they were both very into sports. Rick was two years older than Jessica and was currently at college on a baseball scholarship. It was difficult for Jessica and Rick to be away from each other for so much of the year, but they stayed connected through text messages, video chats, and phone calls.

One evening Rick was late in calling Jessica. They had talked earlier in the day and Jessica told him that she needed him, please call. He said he would make time, but seemed to have lost track of the evening. As the night wore on and Jessica waited for her phone to ring, she grew impatient and angry. It was the first time Jessica was actually angry at Rick. She went to bed angry and hurt that Rick had let her down.

The next morning Jessica awoke to the horrible news that Rick was gone. There had been a car accident and Rick had not survived. Jessica was devastated. And perhaps even worse, she was overcome with tremendous guilt for the anger she'd felt the night before. And over what? Not getting a phone call?! How could she have been so self-absorbed as to not even have considered that something was wrong? Rick had never let her down before – how come she didn't even think to give him the benefit of the doubt? Should she have called him? Would he still be alive today if he'd been on the phone with her? Guilty feelings and self-condemning thoughts plagued Jessica's mind and heart.

Although her first time in residential treatment did not provide a lasting recovery, it did enable Jessica to do some important work that would put her in a better position to succeed the second-go-round. Working with her residential therapist, Jessica began to put her emotional reaction into context. She had not known the whole story upfront. She'd simply been angry because she missed a phone call.

She did not cause Rick's accident and she could not have saved him, either. Her therapist guided her gently down the road to acceptance and forgiveness.

But the breakthrough moment came when Jessica sat among her two best friends in treatment. They helped her write a goodbye letter to Rick. In the letter, Jessica expressed her feelings of anger – not just about him not calling her, but also about him getting into a truck after downing a six pack of beer. She wrote about how angry she was, how guilty she felt, and how much she loved him. When she finished writing, Jessica and her friends cried as Jessica read the letter out loud. Jessica's friends helped her get through the night and by morning she felt as though a weight had been lifted from her. Jessica still missed Rick tremendously, but now when she thought of him, she didn't immediately feel guilt and anger. She felt their love.

 ## Taylor

Today Taylor does not have a close – or even functional – relationship with anyone in her immediate family, but she was close with her mother when she was alive. After Taylor's mother passed away suddenly from pancreatic cancer, she had to cope with the loss of her relationship with her father as well.

"When my mom died, I kind of knew that I had lost both parents," says Taylor. In some ways these losses were related and in some ways they were different. For the last ten years of Taylor's parents' marriage, they experienced marital strife. Taylor became a confidante to her mother, for better and for worse, and as such she heard things about her father that she would not have known otherwise.

"I guess you could say that I went into my relationship with my father with a bias," Taylor explains. Taylor had to grieve the loss of both parents at once. Even though only one of them had died, in reality they were both gone. "It's kind of a weird thing, and I hate to say it, but a lot of times I wish he was actually dead so that I could stop aching and being disappointed by the things he does and doesn't do."

In the last ten years, Taylor's father called her on her birthday only three times. "That's hard," she says, "That hurt doesn't go away."

In order to help herself through the grieving process, Taylor reached out to those closest to her, including her rabbi and his wife, who she describes as "surrogate parents." One of Taylor's greatest strengths lies in her ability to find support. One of the ways she moved past the breakdown of her family was to talk about it to her rabbi and to her friends and to her therapist.

"In terms of my mom," Taylor says, "the biggest thing was letting myself feel whatever I was feeling. And understanding that it was complicated. There were times when I was happy and times when I was sad. And times when they happened at the same time – and that was okay. And I learned to be okay with not having to control that."

Although she admits to using her eating disorder symptoms during this time, Taylor explains that, "My mother was the only thing I have grieved and dealt with in a healthy way. It was the other things in my life that I wasn't dealing with properly." Acting out on her eating disorder, however, did not help her cope with the loss of her relationship with her father. In fact it wasn't until Taylor spent quite some time abstaining from her symptoms that she began to find healing and acceptance.

"I will say that, being in recovery, I am much more accepting of who my father is and what he is able to do, while still acknowledging that he isn't what I need(ed) and that's okay. It has to be okay."

The above stories are stories of grief and loss in the rawest sense. They do not fit into neatly wrapped packages. Loss is an ongoing process that often takes many years. Losing people who are closest to you, or who you wish were closest to you, is terribly painful and requires a lot of courage to face it head on and cope with in a healthy way. In a sense, every person who recovers from an eating disorder goes through a grieving process – grieving the loss of the eating disorder which most likely served as their closest "relationship" during the course of their illness. It takes a lot of strength to move on after a loss. There is no right way to grieve. Every person is different and therefore every person's process is different. Some people find comfort in prayer or in talking to their loved ones who have passed, or in remembering the good times they shared together.

I am close with a family in which the grandfather recently passed away after a lengthy illness. Two of his young grandchildren, an eight-year-old girl and a six-year-old boy, were talking soon after his death. The eight-year-old said, "It makes me so sad when I think about what happened to him."

"Then don't think about what *happened* to him," said the six-year old. "Think about *him*."

Such wisdom!

Just as re-living the painful aspects of loss is counterproductive, after a traumatic incident there also is a real risk of mentally "re-living" the event, or even physically and emotionally recreating it.

For example:

Once while visiting another country I was threatened by a taxicab driver. In order to escape possible danger I had to get away. The driver refused to stop the taxi and drop me off, so while the car was in motion I threw the door open and jumped out. What ensued was severe emotional distress, intense fear of taxis, and eventually anger. I was consumed with thoughts of how I could have handled the situation differently, how I could have called the police or better stood up for myself. I also became hypersensitive to cues of danger, sometimes perceiving danger where it didn't truly exist. On my very next ride in a taxi I once again felt threatened, except that this time the feelings were unwarranted. I began defending myself and threatening to call the police – things I felt I should have done the first time – and in effect *created* a potentially dangerous situation. If this is a pattern that is familiar to you, then you would do well to explore it with a qualified therapist.

Another common theme among those who have experienced trauma, especially at the hands of another person or people, is a feeling or fear of powerlessness. Yet these same individuals who so desperately need to feel safe and secure often spend considerable amounts of time, in therapy and out, in confrontation.

Subconsciously what may be happening is a fabrication of a "second chance" at one's response to the trauma. If you "failed" to say no or to otherwise defend or protect yourself, then you may subconsciously crave a "do-over." This can result in confrontation with therapists, family, friends, and strangers. I strongly suggest that you work to ease up on this type of irrational confrontation not only because it causes added distress, but also because it hinders your healing process. Feelings of powerlessness inside are not resolved by these kinds of external altercations.

Of course you *do* need to stand up for yourself and to protect yourself and to be assertive. How is this done? Through learning to differentiate between "real" and "perceived" threats of danger, and recalibrating your sensitivity to situations in which it is appropriate to exercise assertiveness. Don't make others, including your therapist, mind-read or otherwise decipher your messages. Say what you really mean. Say "no" only when you truly *mean* no. *Make your "no's" count.*

Survivors often question their responses to past traumatic events. Was their response the best? Was there a better solution? Did they do the "right thing?" A professor in my counseling master's degree program stresses that *whatever a survivor does to survive is the right thing.*

As noted earlier, it is important to recognize that while not all traumatic experiences are objectively big "T" traumas, they must still be dealt with appropriately. If a difficult experience has made a lasting negative impact on you, it is considered a trauma. Sometimes people think that because their ordeal was not as severe or earth-shattering as someone else's, it isn't really so bad and that they should just "get over it." Often people with eating disorders, especially upon meeting others in treatment with histories of trauma, wonder why they themselves are experiencing such difficulties when their own lives have been relatively blessed and smooth. This is a mistake.

Just as eating disorders cannot be blamed solely on poor body image or the media, so too they cannot be blamed on trauma. Not everyone who experiences a trauma suffers from an eating disorder and not everyone who suffers from an eating disorder has experienced a trauma. These thoughts are examples of the kind of "black-and-white" thinking that often accompanies eating disorders in the first place.

Taking this faulty need to establish cause and effect out of the picture, it is easier to see more clearly the true effects of certain events on our lives. Sometimes a seemingly mundane occurrence can cause considerable stress. Denying this stress will likely make it harder to heal. Only after acceptance can there be true healing.

❧ Lexi

On February 9, 2004 Lexi slipped on a patch of ice and broke her leg. It is a day that is forever seared into her memory. Prior to this incident, when Lexi thought of broken bones she thought of a month in a cast followed by physical therapy. After that she assumed everything would be back to normal. That's how she'd seen similar situations pan out for others and that's how she assumed hers would work as well. Little did she know her life was about to change.

After being transported to the hospital Lexi learned that she had broken both her tibia and her fibula. *Okay*, she reasoned, *maybe this will be a little worse than I thought, but it still won't be* too *bad.* Lexi remained in the hospital for four days. She was given large amounts of yellow Gatorade – for years the taste and smell of this drink would bring back painful memories. She was also given medications that caused her to forget much of her hospital stay. After her return home, Lexi spent six weeks in a wheelchair, eight weeks on crutches, and another eight weeks in a walking cast. By now she realized that this wasn't simply a broken leg, but she failed to accept that it might have far-reaching consequences.

Lexi was very involved with sports and she wondered how she would ever get back to her original level of performance after breaking her leg. She was unable to play properly for two solid years because of the intense pain in her leg. She lost weight due to all of her medications and her eating disorder began. Lexi lost more than weight, however: She lost her sense of who she was.

When Lexi first began working with a therapist to combat her eating disorder, her therapist asked her repeatedly how she was affected by the trauma of breaking her leg. Lexi denied any long-term effects and refused to consider that a broken leg constituted a "trauma." She told herself, *I know many people with eating disorders who were raped, abused, or lived in alcoholic or drug addicted families – those are* real *traumas. I didn't experience anything even close to those kinds of things, so why do I have an eating disorder?* These thoughts plagued Lexi's mind for a long time as she struggled to make sense of her eating disorder. She was searching for a reason, for validation.

After some time in therapy, Lexi came to the realization that trauma has different meanings. To Lexi it meant any experience that painfully forced her to change the way she thought about herself, or something that she was ashamed of. Her broken leg was more than just a broken bone – it changed what Lexi considered to be her identity. She was no longer a player of collegiate sports. She was ashamed that she could no longer perform at the level she thought others expected of her. She spent many nights crying, wondering what she could possibly do to regain others' praise and approval.

Lexi's therapist taught her a quote: "You are not defined by what you do, but by who you are." This line was repeated to Lexi many times, over and over again, until it sounded like a broken record. It wasn't until Lexi started saying it out loud everyday that she began to believe it. The idea that her performance defined her was deeply ingrained in Lexi's mind. She worked hard in therapy to amend her thoughts. She worked to find the things in life that brought her joy. She spent time being grateful for those activities that she *could* do. She learned to accept this event as a trauma. Just as with other traumas, Lexi had to realize how it changed her life, grieve for what she'd lost, and appreciate what she still had. Lexi had to replace her negativity over how she would never be who she was, with an appreciation for who she *is*.

Lexi now says, "Life is too short to stay stuck in the idea that a past event ruined who you are, because in reality who you are never changes. What changes is what you can become."

Chapter 10

DEVELOPING HEALTHY RELATIONSHIPS

"A friend is someone who understands your past, believes in your future, and accepts you just the way you are."

– Unknown

 Andrew

When his older son lost his hearing and the family thought he might forever be deaf, Andrew was absolutely devastated. (Thankfully he got his hearing back.) When Andrew's younger son almost bled to death from internal injuries, Andrew knew that it wasn't time to have an eating disorder. It was certainly time to be strong for his family, but Andrew learned through his therapy that "no man is an island" and that it is okay – and good – to express feelings.

During these struggles Andrew *was* strong for his family. He *also* cried a lot. One did not contradict the other. Andrew cried on the phone and in people's arms. He accepted that he has needs just like everyone else. He relied on his family and friends for support. But he did *not* rely on any part of the eating disorder.

"My mother says that most people wouldn't have coped so well," says Andrew. "I certainly wasn't going to fall apart and watch my family disintegrate."

Andrew currently does not participate in regular therapy. Because he works as a care worker at the centre at which he was treated, it is easy for him to have a session if he needs it. Andrew feels that he has nipped his eating disorder in the bud, but says that if he ever felt he was slipping then he would go straight back into therapy.

"And actually I didn't need to do that during stress. I feel really good looking back [at the stressful times my family encountered]. The centre doesn't want you to go there forever. They want you to go home and use the skills, to cope with your own life and rely on people in your personal life. Not the eating disorder."

Andrew further explains that when he had an eating disorder he had no relationships. He had almost no desire for relationships. He was overcome with food issues. Andrew also admits that he, in truth, was so *afraid* of relationships because he felt so badly about himself, that he turned to the eating disorder.

The idea that an eating disorder is a relationship is not a new one. Therapists strive to help their clients externalize their problems. The goal is to help a person understand that his or her *problem* is not his or her *identity*. It was out of this externalization that the concept of "Ed" was born. Many people refer to their eating disorders as "Ed" – the initials E.D. standing for "eating disorder." In this way they differentiate between their true identity and the intrusive eating disorder which often seems to have a mind of its own. This personification of the illness ideally serves to drive a separation between the person and his or her eating disorder. In this way one can begin to consciously refute the guidance and input of "Ed" and to live a healthy life. A prime example of this approach runs through the book *Life without Ed*, by Jenni Schaefer.

People struggling with eating disorders can be said to be in an abusive relationship. This isn't to say that the personification *causes* the relationship with "Ed." The relationship was already there, the personification simply shines a clear light on it. Eating disorders are parasitic in nature – they sap their hosts of energy, peace, and love.

Korrie

A turning point in Korrie's recovery came during her high school graduation. Korrie looked around at her fellow graduates – her peers with whom she shared her middle school and high school years. They were happy and smiling, laughing as they took pictures with their friends and families. They reminisced about all the fun they had over the last few years, all the trouble they'd gotten into and all the memories they shared. They discussed their dreams for the rest of their lives and swore to each other they would stay in touch. "Friends forever," they promised. The ceremony began and as each name was called, clapping and cheering filled the auditorium.

Korrie sat alone, feeling left out. When her name was called and it was time for her to publicly receive her diploma, there was no cheering – just silence. Only her family clapped for her because Korrie had no friends. She watched the others in bitter disappointment and regret. Korrie had wasted her middle school and high school years being sick and pushing everyone away. The only thing she had cared about was her eating disorder.

"Being alone was the thing I was most afraid of," Korrie laments, "but in the end that's what the eating disorder did: It made me alone."

When we consider that an eating disorder is an unhealthy coping mechanism it makes sense that to recover we must replace it with healthy coping skills. Therefore it makes sense when we consider an eating disorder as an unhealthy *relationship* that an important factor in recovery is the development of healthy relationships.

An eating disorder is an all-encompassing mess-making machine. It wrecks our bodies, minds, motivation, and just about everything else in our lives – including our relationships. In fact, by destroying our relationships with those closest to us – our friends, families, teachers, and role models – the eating disorder asserts itself as the most important thing in our lives and attempts to replace every relationship we have or need. In this way it "assists" us in losing sight of our true needs and wants and instead leads us to chase imaginary goals. In exchange for our self-destructive behavior, the eating disorder promises us fantastical rewards including warmth, affection, and love. In a moment of blazing honesty we may recognize that the eating disorder can never follow through on such promises. But we *can* have all these things and more through relationships. Real relationships.

Taylor

Because Taylor's family could not meet her needs, she turned to her rabbi and his wife, with whom she had grown close over the years. Taylor began babysitting their daughter when she was thirteen years old and developed a relationship with the family prior to the breakdown of her own family. Even before chaos erupted, Taylor's rabbi, a very intuitive and wise man, was able to see that things were not right within her family and that Taylor was not really being taken care of by anyone. And so, he compassionately took her under his wing.

Most of Taylor's family attended the same synagogue and that was one of the reasons that Taylor confided in him as a teenager. He was able to offer advice in a different way than most because he was able to see more of the picture than most. Very few people understood how destructive Taylor's father was, as he put on a front and presented himself very well in public. He was manipulative and convincing, and very charming. It was sometimes difficult for Taylor to make sense of what went on behind closed doors. People tended to believe him unless they had previously dealt with such people and knew the signs. Taylor's rabbi provided a much needed reality check on many occasions, and served as a healthy father figure to her. He was a shoulder to cry on and was always there to counsel and guide her.

During the winter break of her sophomore year of college, Taylor went back home to stay with her biological father. However, after a huge fight broke out, she called her rabbi and asked plainly, "Can I come and stay with you?" He said yes.

From then on it was somehow understood that whenever Taylor was in town, she would stay with the rabbi and his wife, who she came to view as surrogate parents. She trusted them, in large part due to their counseling roles in the community. At a certain point, Taylor did a family therapy session with her rabbi, which helped give her therapist a better sense of the situation.

Eventually for her own wellbeing Taylor had to cut ties with her father. She stopped taking his phone calls and refused to discuss him with other members of her extended family. There were times that he tried to see her, but Taylor steeled herself against what she knew would be destructive interactions. It was, and still is, painful. But it is necessary in order for her to move on and live a happy, healthy life.

Taylor continues to feel at home with her rabbi's family. They may not be blood relatives, but they *are* her family. They help her through difficult times and celebrate with her in good times. The rabbi's wife cheered for her at her college graduation. While it hurt that her father wasn't in attendance, Taylor was grateful that her "adopted" family was. As she received her degree, Taylor looked on into the audience and knew she was loved.

I didn't fully understand the healing nature of relationships with others in recovery until very recently when, after a difficult therapy session, I called up a couple of friends for support. I was struggling with some news I'd been given earlier that day – my therapist told me that my "mood swings" were often more than just your run-of-the-mill mood swings and that, in her opinion, I struggled with certain aspects of bipolar. We even went through the diagnostic criteria for bipolar and together determined that, yes; the issues involved were eerily similar to my own.

After I left the session I felt conflicted. On the one hand I *hated* the idea that I could be even remotely bipolar. But on the other hand, it did seem to make sense in the context of my emotional struggles. I thought about it, stewed about it, internally debated about it. The next day I called a recovery friend. She was out with another one of our friends and I went to meet up with them. I knew they would be supportive, I knew they would understand, I knew they would commiserate and tell me that everything would be okay…

"What's the matter?" they asked me.

"My therapist thinks I struggle with issues similar to bipolar," I said nervously.

"So what?" they asked, unimpressed.

So what?!

"Excuse me?" I was not happy with this flip little attitude of theirs.

"So what that she thinks that?" one of them added, "'bipolar' is just a word, a label. It doesn't *mean* anything about who you are or anything." She went on to tell me that at one point she was diagnosed bipolar but different doctors had different opinions about it. Some said she was bipolar, others said that's ridiculous. The diagnosis of these things is irrelevant a lot of the time, she told me. It doesn't mean anything is different than how you were before the diagnosis was made. The words just give you something to work with, but they don't define who you *are.*

Our other friend piped in, "That word, 'bipolar' – it doesn't mean you're part of a club! It's the same as an eating disorder. You don't join some secret society by being sick. Sick doesn't mean special. Sick just means sick."

Put in that way I was able to differentiate between myself and my struggles. No longer would I allow myself to be chained up or dragged down by these words. I began using the words to help me fight the problem. Now that I know the nature of some of my struggles I can face them in a more real way. I felt empowered and it was thanks to my recovery friends. I always knew that they could be there for me and understand me. But until this point I didn't realize how much they could challenge me (in a good way!) sometimes even more than any of my therapists or nutritionists or doctors of any kind.

That's one side of the coin. Recovery friends can be extremely helpful, challenging, and supportive. But what happens when they are not? What about situations in which one or both friends begin to slip or offer less-than-helpful "guidance?" How do you maintain (or break away from) the relationship? How do you maintain healthy boundaries?

Korrie

Alison was the first person Korrie befriended after leaving treatment. Alison had recently lost a lot of weight, and she seemed to Korrie to be pretty and skinny and perfect. Korrie reflects that during that time in her life she attracted "sick people" and that her relationship with Alison was no different. "Our relationship wasn't healthy," says Korrie.

Korrie and Alison engaged in a lot of unspoken competition. Alison always seemed to have "won" and Korrie was left feeling second best. Alison continually hogged the spotlight, it seemed. Over time Alison became sicker and sicker. Korrie eventually took a step back from the friendship.

A year later Alison went into treatment herself and contacted Korrie upon her release, saying that she was better and that "treatment changed her life." Alison was extremely convincing and Korrie decided to give the friendship another chance. Korrie was unsure about getting involved in a potentially "toxic" situation, but she reasoned that Alison had a good heart and Korrie liked her and cared about her a lot. Korrie also realized that she was much more self-aware than she had been when they first became friends. Korrie felt stronger now, much healthier.

Indeed, Korrie was healthier and more self-aware. After two weeks passed, she understood that her friendship with Alison was still toxic. Alison was still very sick and manipulative. The familiar old patterns of competition began to emerge once more. Nevertheless Korrie tried to stick it out and be there for her friend. Several weeks later Korrie's feelings of hurt and anger and frustration built up until she felt she would burst. She finally confronted Alison and told her that they could not be friends anymore. There were no expletives, but Korrie was certain and firm.

At this point Korrie knew that she'd come a long way. It took a lot of inner strength and courage to end the friendship and move on. Alison was special to Korrie but there came a time when Korrie realized that she'd been holding on to the friendship for unhealthy reasons. Alison was extremely social, a people pleaser. And she hardly ever said no. Alison did not show her true self. She always had to be "perfect" and liked by others. Korrie, on the other hand, was more assertive. She let her feelings show – she wasn't always happy and peppy. She realized that for precisely this reason she could never win against Alison.

And that's when Korrie began to appreciate that true friendship is not a competition. It's not about who is better, stronger, prettier, thinner... it's about two people who care about each other and are there for one another as equals. Korrie perpetually felt like Alison's caretaker as she tried to protect her from illness and poor decisions. Korrie still wanted to help Alison, but no matter how sad she was for Alison and no matter how much she tried to help, things did not improve. When the friendship reached a point where it was not only unhelpful to Alison but also harmful to Korrie, it had to be broken off. In the end, Korrie knew she had to take care of herself and that the only one who could help Alison... was Alison.

Jen Nardozzi cautions that maintaining relationships formed with other people in treatment can be tricky. "It can be very hard if someone you're friends with is stumbling and you yourself are still trying to get steady," she says. Jen describes the early stages of recovery as "Bambi Legs" – when a baby deer (like Disney's Bambi) is born, its legs are wobbly and unsteady. It takes time and practice for the young deer to strengthen its legs to walk steadily.

"When you had the structure of treatment it is okay," she continues, "but then when the container is taken away it's difficult," especially when one or both friends are experiencing the ups and downs of recovery. Jen advises her clients to be cognizant of their level of ability to help others – the balance between helping others and remaining strong themselves. If helping another person will put your recovery at risk, it is generally best to take care of yourself first. If you feel guilty about this, then consider the following: If you do not take care of yourself, first and foremost, and wind up compromising your own wellbeing, then you will be less able to help others in the future.

People who struggle with eating disorders tend to be people who are caring, supportive, and helpful, but you have to be aware of how much help you can reasonably provide. It is a common occurrence for two recovery friends to begin slipping simultaneously. The closer they get, the more they both struggle. It can be hard to pull back and acknowledge that a friendship is no longer healthy or in the best interest of either party, but in the long run it is sometimes what must be done. Until you can help yourself, you are unable to truly help another person.

Healthy relationships with other people begin with healthy relationships with ourselves. Until we can take proper care of ourselves we will be hard-pressed to engage in positive relationships with others. The boundaries that exist in friendships, romance, and all other relationships must be present in our relationships with ourselves. For example, we need to regularly take time away from our daily routines and set it aside for ourselves. Relationships naturally fizzle out if two people don't spend enough time together. It's the same with our self-relationships.

We have to take "me time." For me, "Naomi time" consists of anything from relaxing on the beach to journaling to random fun activities that I make up on the spot. I recently discovered the wonder that is www.youtube.com and began creating short videos. I also realized that I can write my own music and record it without any musical instruments. I do this by recording several layers of myself singing "do-do-do" such that I am essentially harmonizing with myself. Even if no one ever hears my music, it's a fun way to express myself creatively and blow off steam after a long, busy day.

In addition to spending time with ourselves, we must nurture our intuition. Jen Nardozzi calls this "listening from the inside out."

"It's good to have downtime – whatever that means for you, whether that means walking, meditating, or any other quiet activity," she says, explaining that certain patterns begin to emerge as these activities become a regular part of your life. "You begin to know what you like, what comes up for you in the quiet. You learn what you need and that the answers really are within you. By connecting in this way you can hear the wisdom of your own soul – the quiet voice within." This should give you a clearer direction in terms of knowing how to better care for yourself in body, mind, and spirit. Ask yourself the deeper questions in life – don't be afraid to "go there." What fulfills you? What helps you feel connected, and are you engaging in those things?

Aurora

For a long time, Aurora constantly wanted to be in an intimate, romantic relationship. She thought that if only she had a boyfriend then she would find happiness and feel whole again after the terrible losses she suffered. She needed others, it seemed, to define her and to give her meaning and direction. She got involved in an unhealthy relationship in which she was taken advantage of and made to feel inadequate. In ending and healing from that relationship, Aurora became more in touch with her own self and her own drives and passions.

"I learned what I want for myself," she says. At first it was difficult for her to develop her identity independent of a significant other. After some time she was able to rediscover her true self and connect with her inner power. For Aurora this was a process that had to take place on her own. She took time off from dating seriously in order to focus on herself and her recovery. "That isn't to say that I wouldn't go on a date here and there," she says, "but I was very selective about who I allowed myself to get involved with." Aurora also notes that contrary to past negative experiences, her time spent refocusing gave her the strength and perspective to recognize warning signs and act on them.

"If I feel that [a relationship] is in any way unhealthy then I get out of there," she says. "It was a *big* step for me to learn how to do that. It's a milestone for me to say that I can recognize when a dating relationship is unhealthy for me and learn to get out, to use my voice, to tell guys 'no.' It's really empowering to be able to have that ability to make that choice to say I won't be living up to someone else's standards of approval. I don't live to make others happy. I have to be happy on my own before I can be happy with someone else."

Boundaries are part and parcel of healthy relationships. In Chapter 2 boundaries were discussed as they relate to therapeutic relationships. In truth they are crucial to *all* relationships. As in Aurora's case, it is important to be a whole person yourself before connecting with others. Rather than considering yourself half a person searching for your other half, consider that you are already a whole person. You don't need anyone to complete you. Of course we need others in our lives, but we cannot be so dependent on others that we can't function on our own. Only after developing yourself and your own identity can you properly love another person. This is true not only of romantic relationships, but also of relationships with friends, family, co-workers, and others. Healthy boundaries are a must.

Jen Nardozzi recommends, "Start noticing how you are feeling when you're with this person. Are you feeling drained? Are you more worried about that person than about your own wellbeing? Does it feel like too much? Like you're doing therapy with this person? Notice how *you're* doing – ask yourself, 'am I going beyond my boundaries by using all of my helping energy on other people and leaving little for myself?' Continue to check in with yourself."

Recovery friends are certainly important, but it's *extremely* important to make sure that your relationship is based upon more than eating disorders. If eating disorders and recovery are all you ever talk about, then there's a good chance that the relationship will slide into the realm of unhealthy and unhelpful. Even then, there are ways to keep yourself in a good place.

"Relationships in treatment are really important because they mimic, and often take on, the form of a person's relationships outside and also their family dynamics," says Rebekah Bardwell Doweyko. "The treatment team tends to be more like 'Mom and Dad' but your relationships with others in recovery take on a dynamic similar to what it's like on the outside." It's an opportunity to practice doing things differently in recovery than what you may have done previously that didn't serve you well in the past.

Rebekah explains that these friendships are helpful so long as both parties are doing well in their recovery. When one person is going strong and the other begins to struggle, it makes continuing the relationship in a healthy way very difficult. The friend who is not struggling may *begin* to struggle as the relationship wears on, since eating disorders tend to become competitive in nature. If you begin to struggle because of your friendship with someone who is struggling, then you would do well to consider taking a step back from the relationship, or even discontinuing it completely.

Be honest with yourself about your ability to manage the boundaries in such a friendship. If you've been in recovery for a long time and honestly know in your heart that you are not being negatively affected, then it is possible to continue the relationship. But if at any point you are negatively impacted, it may be time to reconsider. Things for which you should be on the lookout include control imbalances and acting out of fear of losing a friend. It's also important that both friends look outside the friendship for additional support.

"Being a real friend to somebody who starts to struggle means not enabling their relapse," says Rebekah. Continuing the friendship at the same level basically communicates to your struggling friend that relapse is okay and, no matter what, you will remain friends – no consequences. Although it is difficult, setting boundaries at such a time is actually the greatest thing you can do for your friend. Rebekah suggests the simple sentiment, "I love you, I care about you, and I want to be your friend more than anything. But I can't be your friend and your eating disorder's friend." Explain that they do not need to be perfect, but that they must make the effort to turn things around.

Jen Nardozzi advises that if a friend, particularly a recovery friend, begins relying on you too much, it is beneficial to set more explicit boundaries and insist that they be honored. It is appropriate and okay to tell a friend that you can't be available for them day or night. If you are not emotionally available at any given time, for whatever reason, be honest about it and say that you are unable to help at that time rather than push yourself past your healthy limits. You don't have to leave your friend hanging, but you can say that it may be better if you both pick another time to talk. "Healing occurs within relationships. When people create healthy relationships with themselves and with others, then they don't need the eating disorder anymore. Thus, healthy relationships are key in recovery." It's all about boundaries.

These are important issues for everyone, not only those in recovery from eating disorders. Relationships are part of healthy living. Everyone – yes everyone – struggles from time to time with boundaries in relationships. This can mean anything from an extreme lack of boundaries to a more subtle worry about "why am I the only one who ever calls so-and-so to make plans?" Jen recommends taking stock of your relationships from time to time. And never underestimate the value of "gut feelings." If someone or some situation gives you a "bad vibe," listen to yourself and trust your intuition. Rebekah Bardwell Doweyko cautions that "if a person is not emotionally well, then they're not going to get the most intuitive gut feelings." However, there is no need to despair. Issues can be resolved, emotional health can be attained and boundaries can be learned.

Balance. Are your relationships balanced? Are you always giving? Are you always taking? Suggestions for bettering relationships in which you are always giving are discussed above. But what about if you find yourself always taking?

Jen Nardozzi suggests that if you feel that you are always taking, you may first want to check it out. There's nothing wrong with directly asking the question. Request feedback from the other person or people. You can phrase it in a gentle way, such as "I'm going through a hard time and I know I'm coming to you a lot – is that okay?" There is a chance you truly *are* taking too much, but there is also a chance that you are sensitive about being a burden on others, especially if you feel that has been a pattern in your life due to your eating disorder or other difficulties. Or perhaps, on the contrary, you were always a giving person who always put others first and your self-image is based on those qualities. Asking for support for yourself can feel uncomfortable and vulnerable. Therapists are a great resource in improving the quality of your relationships – both for those in recovery from eating disorders and for those who have never experienced an eating disorder in their lives.

Chapter 11

PREPARING FOR THE JOURNEY AHEAD

"Every day brings something new and
challenging… face it head on."

– Taylor

I was baking cookies with my sister Adina. Adina is an extremely
talented baker and, you could say, I still have a thing or two to
learn. Adina made the dough and was shaping the cookies on
the pan. My one and only job was to drop spoonfuls of cookie
dough into a bowl of flour. As you can probably imagine, this
was not the most exciting job on the planet and I got bored. I
started eating cookie dough and my sister asked me to stop and
go wash my hands. (Isn't she *bossy*?) Meanwhile I got distracted;
I helped myself to a different snack and then went to check my
email. When I returned to the kitchen I was greeted by my less-
than-amused sister.

"Is *focus* one of your coping skills?" she quipped. "Because
you clearly haven't mastered that one yet."

There is always more to learn and room to grow. In the
very beginning, when I was learning to lead a healthy life after
treatment, recovery seemed to be solely about food and staying
healthy. I have since discovered that part of the reason recovery

is an ongoing process is that there is so much more to learn than just nutrition facts. Recovery means living an authentically healthy life. It is about maturity and growth. Recovery is not a perfect linear progression. There will be ups and downs. Recovery is about knowing how to pull through challenges and keep going strong.

But just as it is important to keep improving and growing, it is equally important to reflect on your progress and celebrate your successes, big and little. Successes are more than just the events or actions themselves. They are about the thoughts, feelings, and meanings that we ascribe to them. Take the following story of a cocktail dress…

Korrie

Her high school graduation was rapidly approaching and teenaged Korrie went shopping with her mother for a new dress. Korrie tried on several dresses and none seemed quite right until she found a stunning cocktail dress. She put it on and she immediately loved it. The salespeople complimented her, saying she looked great. For a girl who'd struggled for so long and so intensely against negative body image, this was a moment of bliss.

Then her mother remarked that the dress was unflattering and in fact made her look fat.

Korrie was devastated. How could her *mother* say such a thing to her?! For the first time, Korrie considered that her mother was currently the one with distorted body image. Usually such a comment – especially coming from her mother – would mean that Korrie wouldn't buy the dress, but today was different. Today Korrie was stronger. She realized that the first thing she had done upon putting on the dress was look at her mother's face to gauge how good she looked in it. Why?

Korrie looked in the mirror again. She looked more like a woman than a little girl and she liked it. She wondered if maybe that was the same reason that her mother *didn't* like the dress. Maybe it was difficult for her mother to see her growing up? Korrie bought the dress. It was hard for her to go against her mother's advice and she felt slightly guilty about it. But at the same time, this was *Korrie's* graduation and it was up to *Korrie* to decide what to wear!

Graduation was hard because Korrie felt so isolated from her peers. But she didn't take it out on her body image. In fact, she felt terrific in her new dress. She finally realized that her isolation had nothing to do with how she looked or how her dress looked. It had to do with her eating disorder and how she had pushed everyone away. The loneliness and hurt was the worst she'd ever felt. At that moment she was motivated to change. The experience catapulted Korrie to new heights in therapy. She began talking about real issues. She came to understand that her social struggles were not about her specific friends, teachers, or family members. These patterns repeated *throughout* her life and with *everyone* in her life. It was up to Korrie to change.

In her new cocktail dress Korrie caught a glimpse of herself as a mature woman. And as she wore the dress at graduation, she began to grow into her adult self.

Recovery is also about the understanding that not every issue or challenge is unique to you or to people with eating disorders. I know someone whose daughter underwent residential treatment for her eating disorder and soon afterwards went away to college. This woman told her nervous daughter, "Now you are just as messed up as everyone else in the dorms, but *you* have better *coping skills*."

A common theme among those struggling with eating disorders and other addictive behaviors is the erroneous belief that one must constantly be entertained, happy, or otherwise engaged in exciting activities. Faulty thinking associated with this belief leads people to sensation-seeking behaviors that promise to provide stimulation and excitement. This includes dangerous thrill-seeking behaviors and engagement in interpersonal drama, or drama surrounding eating disorders and other illnesses.

(Some thrill-seeking (or high-seeking) behaviors are more subtle. As you may recall, we discussed in Chapter 5 that a change in the taste of food may indicate fullness. Prior to becoming aware of this phenomenon, I sought that "first high" – the first bite tasted so good and I wanted that back. I kept thinking, "Maybe this bite will be better!" I overate that way. It wasn't until my therapist pointed it out to me that I realized what I had been doing.)

Some of the best moments are downtime moments – moments simply of peace and quiet. Perhaps no one knows this better than Taylor:

℘ Taylor

Taylor used to seek out the excitement around her. She thrived, it seemed, on action. As long as there was something going on, there was something to write about, share with others – something interesting about which to regale friends. Then one evening Taylor sat alone in her room reflecting on her recent experiences. She wanted to write – but, about what? There seemed to be nothing noteworthy. So she wrote a piece about that and it led to an understanding about life and a contentment she hadn't experienced in years, if ever:

"Not Much to Report" was the title. "I was talking to a dear friend of mine recently about communication I'd just had with my father. She asked when the last time we spoke was, and I told her it had been almost a year. She paused – shocked – then asked if it had really been that long. It seemed like she and I had just talked about him coming back into my life. I realized something at that point, but thought I'd take it one step further. I asked if she had a guess as to how long it had been since I moved into my apartment. When I told her it had been almost ten months, she was, again, shocked.

"What occurred to me is that the reason these events seemed so recent to many of my friends, is that my life has been incredibly stable over the past year. Prior to that – whether of my own doing or not – my life was chaotic. I always had one fire or another to put out – so those often acted as time markers for the people in my life. Whether I was mourning a previous loss, suffering a new loss, getting a job, losing a job, changing jobs, going into or out of treatment – there was always something going on. For the past fifteen years of my life, I'm not sure I'd gone more than six months without a major change or crisis. My life was exhausting for me, but it was equally exhausting for the people closest to me. Granted, I wasn't always dealt the best hand. It seemed that if something bad was going to happen, it was probably going to happen to me. But that's no longer true.

"I worked incredibly hard to get myself to my current position. I had difficult, painful conversations with people, often repeatedly advocating for myself when it was the last thing I wanted to or felt worthy of doing. I decided that

I was no longer willing to be the victim all the time, and I made choices about where I was going to live, how I was going to get there, and how to live my daily life. The interesting thing is that this year has not been without change; in fact, quite the opposite. In 2010, I moved into my own apartment, ended a toxic relationship with my former roommate, got a new job, started and ended romantic relationships, traveled, and worked to get myself out of my financial hole. Every day brings something new and challenging, and I face it head on. All told, however, not much is going on – and I'm starting to get used to that being an amazing and empowering thing. So – not much to report…"

While I wouldn't say the best news is no news, I *would* say that the best news tends to be the kind that doesn't make headlines!

As you progress in your recovery you will undoubtedly be presented with more and more opportunities to help others, in a sense coming full circle. Taking advantage of these opportunities and contributing to the wellbeing of other people helps not only them, but you as well. We as humans naturally benefit from being kind and giving. It keeps us on the straight and narrow and enhances our own wellbeing. In fact, the twelfth step of 12-step fellowships is carrying the message of recovery to others.

Andrew

Sitting across from Andrew in the café was a woman named Stephanie. She was a care worker from Marino Therapy Centre, the outpatient clinic at which Andrew ultimately recovered from his eating disorder. Care workers functioned differently than therapists in that they were not trained to do actual therapy. Instead, they were people from the community who were recovered from eating disorders themselves who gave back to others by way of spending time with them in a healthy, structured way. Of course they also collaborated with the client's treatment team, and Andrew knew about this and agreed to it.

Stephanie took Andrew out into the world to do regular things like visiting art galleries and eating out at restaurants. Today they sat in a very popular café sipping coffee. It was a first step towards a healthy life for Andrew in a number of ways.

First of all, it was a chance for Andrew to overcome his great fear of eating in public. Today was the first time he got a cup of coffee at a café. Later on he would work his way up to eating snacks in public and meals at restaurants.

While Stephanie engaged Andrew in conversation, Andrew looked around the café and observed others eating. He thought to himself that he would never be able to do it. Stephanie asked Andrew about his plans and ambitions.

"Most of my ambitions at that moment were body related and unreasonable," Andrew recalls. "I wanted to put on weight, to be muscular. I hated being skinny so I hid away from society as much as I could."

But Andrew had other goals as well. He wanted to get married, have kids, and overcome his social anxiety. Stephanie listened patiently to Andrew's talk of body image goals and responded positively, noting only the emotions and optimism that Andrew expressed.

"She couldn't say, 'Great – hit the gym!' That's not fair," says Andrew. But she did validate his feelings and experience and that was very therapeutic and beneficial for Andrew. Care working is client-directed. Andrew could use it for anything that he wanted. He chose to use it to break out of his shell.

Prior to recovery all Andrew had was an eating disorder. No relationships. After recovery he had a family. Andrew points back to his days working with Stephanie as the building blocks that led him to where he is now, socially. He decided to give back as well, using his experience to help others. Now he is a care worker like Stephanie.

"I found care working brilliant when I was in the program so I decided to do it too."

When Andrew sees someone who is struggling with an eating disorder, he often wishes he could go over to them and help.

"I'm grateful that I'm no longer in that position and my heart goes out to them. I wish they'd get the right kind of help. I understand that you can't just walk up to these people and tell them what they need to do because you'll freak them out," says Andrew. But he still wishes to help in some way, and so he gives back through care working.

Many people believe that after experiencing hardship, it is beneficial to both themselves and others for them to actively help people going through similar struggles. While it is not your job to "save the world," it is *absolutely* your job to do your part.

In Chapter 8 the concept of finding meaning in struggles was explored. It is very common for those who have experienced the pain and struggles of an eating disorder to develop a passion for helping others. Perhaps you or someone you know wants to become a therapist or motivational speaker or in some other form use personal experiences to help others suffering from eating disorders. These are lofty goals but they are not the only ways to make sense of your struggle or to achieve your dream of helping others.

Oftentimes people will share their stories of recovery with others in the hope of inspiring them toward their own recoveries or to participate in eating disorder awareness or advocacy programs.

Participation, for some, is a helpful tool both for themselves and others. For others it can be not only unhelpful but even harmful. It is important to have a certain degree of self-understanding in order to ascertain whether or not these activities are for you.

Your decision to either participate or refrain from such activities is entirely up to you and in no way reflects on the quality of your recovery or your desire to help others. It is simply a matter of personal choice.

Lexi

Mentoring had always been a significant part of Lexi's life. She volunteered with Big Brothers Big Sisters, tutored younger students in school, and spent time talking to and connecting with the teenagers in her church's youth program. Helping others and giving of her time provided Lexi with a sense of meaning and fulfillment.

When she was stable enough in her own recovery, Lexi took up involvement with an online support group for those in recovery from eating disorders. She became a mentor to a young woman battling anorexia. Lexi had originally joined the online group in order to support others and to give back in a simple, predetermined way. Soon, however, Lexi found that the unconditional love, acceptance, and understanding she received from other members on the site was changing her life and building her self-confidence. She decided to take a more active role in the support site and create a recovery group specifically for teenagers. That was when she met her mentee, a beautiful young woman named Tina with whom Lexi instantly connected.

Lexi and Tina decided on one rule from the very beginning: Honesty at all times. In the world of eating disorders there are lies and deceitful behaviors. "Honesty is power" became their motto as together they traveled down Tina's unknown road of recovery. Lexi helped Tina find a local treatment team and encouraged her to attend her appointments. She continues to help Tina differentiate between the voice of her eating disorder, which they call "Ed," and Tina's own voice. Lexi finds it extremely rewarding to see Tina grow spiritually and emotionally. Tina is learning to find herself outside of her eating disorder and is coming to realize that while holding on to her eating disorder she cannot attain her true goals.

As for Lexi, the relationship is a great asset to her own recovery. It gives her a reason to stay on the right path during difficult times when her natural instinct is to go back to using symptoms. Lexi wants to lead a congruent life, to "practice what she preaches." She is grateful for Tina for allowing her into her life, for sharing so much with her, and for giving her a sense of purpose. The honesty rule does more than keep Tina in line – it keeps Lexi on the straight and narrow too. In working together for the shared goal of advanced recovery, Lexi and Tina courageously and honestly confront their challenges and are coming to accept that no one is perfect, nor should they be. In fact, it is precisely our flaws that make us beautiful and unique.

Helping other people through your own experience is something you would do well to carefully consider before jumping in. The first thing to consider is whether it will help or harm your own recovery. It is not your job to save the world. If you are not ready or willing to share your story publicly or with any particular person, do not allow yourself to be pressured into compliance. This goes not only for the beginning stages of recovery but also for any time when you don't feel comfortable sharing or being involved in the world of eating disorders.

If and when you decide you are comfortable and ready to use your eating disorder experience to give back, through writing or speaking or mentoring for example, there are a few guidelines to follow:

- *Know what you are comfortable sharing ahead of time.* Just because you are sharing your story doesn't mean you have to share *everything*. Mentally review your experience and decide upon your personal boundaries of sharing. Practice ways to politely decline questions outside of these boundaries. A simple, "I'm not comfortable sharing that," or "I'd like to keep that private," can do the trick. Rest assured that people will respect your boundaries.

- *Avoid triggering information.* This includes numbers pertaining to weights, calories, and clothing sizes. You should also avoid going into too much detail regarding symptom usage. Especially when speaking with teenagers and young adults, there is the risk of "teaching" vulnerable listeners how to have an eating disorder. In addition, those who may be struggling already – or even those in recovery – may be drawn towards comparing themselves, their symptoms, and numbers, with yours. This is dangerous in two ways: First, someone may decide that because your numbers and symptoms are different than theirs that means they are not "sick enough." They may increase their own symptom use as a result of this faulty thinking. Second, someone may interpret the difference in numbers or symptoms to mean that they really are not so bad off after all. This thinking can aid their denial and prevent them from seeking treatment. It's a good idea to emphasize that all eating disorders are dangerous, regardless of the specific symptoms and numbers involved, and that everyone who struggles deserves treatment and support.

- *Know your audience and tailor your information to suit their needs.* A group of high school students has different needs than a group of parents of teenagers, and both have different needs than a group of individuals actively battling eating disorders. Sharing your story publicly is not about *you*; it is about your *message*.

- *Contemplate risks and rewards.* Consider the potential impact of what you wish to say to your audience; not only to the attendees, but also to yourself. While there is certainly the possible reward that you will feel good about helping others, there is also the possible risk that you will feel exposed and wish you could take back some, or all, of what you said – especially if you did not take the time to determine your boundaries beforehand.

Not everyone can, or should, use their personal eating disorder experience as a direct means of helping others. Especially in the beginning stages of recovery it can be difficult to differentiate between your own experience and others' experiences. What helped you may not help other people. When you aim to help others overcome their challenges, it must be about the other person, not about you. This can be a serious struggle if eating disorders hit too close to home. There are other ways to give back. Use your strengths, interests, and talents to make a difference.

 ## Korrie

Korrie does not use her personal story of recovery as a direct means with which to help others. After one negative speaking experience, she feels she now has a well-balanced approach to sharing her story.

During a period of recovery between two relapses, Korrie was asked to share her story at a conference. She agreed and spoke alongside others who shared educative information and personal stories about eating disorders. Although she had been feeling fairly strong at the start, she now admits that she was not ready to participate in such an event. Sharing her story at the conference brought up all the emotions and the pain of her eating disorder and Korrie was not prepared. She began to struggle more and more intensely as time elapsed after the conference, eventually spiraling into a full-blown relapse.

Working hard with her outpatient team, Korrie revitalized her recovery. With her deepened self-awareness, she recognized that sharing her story was not the avenue by which she was comfortable helping others. If she feels her story can help another person, and that she herself can communicate it in a healthy and helpful way, she sometimes considers sharing it privately in a one-on-one discussion. But in general she does not "bend over backwards" to find opportunities to share her story.

"I don't want to be known as the girl who had an eating disorder," says Korrie. "I can help people in other ways. I coach gymnastics, I teach in a preschool. I do those things to help the kids."

At the age of eighteen, Korrie discovered an important truth. The meaning in her struggle and her resulting desire to help others and contribute to society can be actualized in a number of different ways. Today Korrie is considering her options as she will soon begin her college career.

"I know I want to do something meaningful that helps people," she says, but she also recognizes that nearly every field has the potential to better the lives of others.

It can be tempting to think that in order to make a difference things need to be a certain way. For instance, you might think that you need to have an advanced degree or be in a position of influence in order to impact other people. Nothing is farther from the truth. You can – and always *do* – influence others with your actions.

I recently saw a very powerful scene in the popular television show *House* illustrating this point. Dr. House is a prominent diagnostician who suffers from a drug addiction. After a long, drawn-out battle, he grudgingly agrees to go into treatment. Dr. House breaks the rules and tries every scheme he can imagine to get out of the psychiatric ward on which he finds himself living. Through his defiance he becomes a hero to his roommate, a bipolar man who refuses to take his medication or take any strides towards achieving wellness. Near the end of the show, Dr. House complies with his treatment program and his distraught roommate quips, "They broke you!"

"No," responds Dr. House. "They didn't break me. I'm already broken." He then proceeds to follow the rules and slowly he begins to heal. His roommate soon watches him through the window as he is discharged from the ward and allowed to return to his life outside the hospital walls. Afterwards, the roommate walks to the nurse's station.

"What do you need?" a nurse asks him.

"My medicine," the man replies. "I want to get better."

Through his example, Dr. House impacted his roommate's life, possibly setting him on the path to recovery and wellness. As I watched this episode I was stuck by the realization that no matter where a person may be, the power to influence always remains. You may be a teacher in a school or a leader of an organization or a patient in a clinic. We discussed in Chapter 3 that some roles are transient and others are more permanent, but the true self remains the same. This includes the ability to help others. Think about it. How many times have you been influenced by the words or actions of another person? How often has a hug or a kind gesture gotten you through a difficult moment? One simple smile can brighten a person's day. If you have ever been positively impacted by another person, you must by definition believe in your own power to make a difference.

Lexi

After years of recovery, Lexi relapsed. One slip led to another and before she knew it, things had spiraled out of her control. She had always been one to support the claim that people can and do recover on an outpatient basis. And while that remains true, Lexi swallowed her pride and checked herself into a residential treatment facility far from home. After several weeks she was back in an outpatient setting, where she continued working hard in order to reclaim her recovery and her life. During her relapse she lost nearly everything – her school, her close relationships, her position as a mentor, and so on. It took a lot for her to gain it all back, but Lexi was determined.

She also never gave up. Not on herself and not on others. Throughout her struggles, she plastered her Facebook wall with inspirational quotes and encouragement to her friends and loved ones.

At the time of my writing this publication Lexi was still in outpatient treatment. She asked me once if that meant she could no longer share her story in the book. My response? Her story was now even *more* important to the book! Lexi is a shining example of strength and responsibility. She had the integrity to seek help and to work hard. She never took treatment for granted. Just before she entered residential treatment she expressed to me how fortunate she felt to have the opportunity. Not everyone is so lucky. She's right. If you are fortunate enough to have resources to help you – no matter what they are or how frustrating you find them – cherish them. Use them well. And work hard. You are blessed with opportunity.

Although it should be obvious by now, it is still worth spelling out that *there will be struggles in recovery.* Sometimes little struggles and sometimes big struggles. A slip doesn't equal a relapse. When you slip or struggle the best thing is to just get up and keep going. Do the next right thing. There is no use giving up or catastrophizing or throwing a pity party. Take a moment to refocus your energy and move on. The people sharing their stories throughout this book provide strong examples of proactive recovery.

When you think back over the stories of recovery in this book, who do you see? You could easily lump them all together and see them as people in recovery from eating disorders. By now it is more likely that you see them as distinctive individuals, each with different drives and passions, hopes and dreams. They are certainly more than their respective eating disorders or weights or exercise habits. They are more than their failings and they are more than their pasts. They are valuable people who make the world better through their unique contributions to society – to their communities, families, and friends. They each have the potential to live whatever life they choose, and to achieve brilliant success as they define it. And guess what? So can you.

You keep doing well because you keep doing what works – using your skills, your support system, and your treatment team. You have the insight, you have the skills. You know what to do. Recover your life and achieve your dreams because, in essence, recovery is not about the illness that *was* – it's about the life that *is*.

Useful Contacts

The author can be contacted at nfeigenbaum@gmail.com.

The contact details of the treatment centers discussed in this book are listed below.

The Renfrew Centers

Telephone: +1 (800) RENFREW

Website: www.renfrewcenter.com

The centers provide a comprehensive range of services in nine states: Pennsylvania, Florida, New York City, Connecticut, New Jersey, North Carolina, Tennessee, Texas, and Maryland.

Center for Intuitive Eating

Telephone: +1 (800) 403 4208

Website: www.hollywoodpavilion.com

Treatment is provided in a community of empowerment, healing, respect, compassion, and growth.

The Cleveland Center for Eating Disorders (CCED)

Telephone: +1 (216) 765 0500

Website: www.edcleveland.com

The center is committed to providing effective treatment for children, adolescents, and adults suffering from eating disorders.

Marino Therapy Centre

Telephone: +353 1 833 3126

Website: www.marinotherapycentre.com

Marino Therapy Centre (in Dublin, Ireland) has over fifteen years' experience successfully helping sufferers of eating disorders (both men and women) to fully recover and live their lives free from the eating distress condition.

Further Reading

Conry, B.M (2001) *Believe in Yourself* (mini book). New York, NY: Peter Pauper Press.

David, M. (1994) *Nourishing Wisdom: A Mind-Body Approach to Nutrition and Well-Being*. New York, NY: Three Rivers Press.

Johnston, A. (2000) *Eating in the Light of the Moon: How Women can Transform their Relationship with Food through Myths, Metaphors & Storytelling*. Carlsbad, CA: Gürze Books.

Linehan, M.M. (1993) *Cognitive Behavioral Treatment for Borderline Personality Disorder*. New York, NY: Guilford Publications.

Linehan, M.M. (1993) *Skills Training Manual for Treating Borderline Personality Disorder*. New York, NY: Guilford Publications.

Satter, E. (2008) *Secrets of Feeding a Healthy Family: How to Eat, How to Raise Good Eaters, How to Cook*. Madison, WI: Kelcy Press. See also www.ellynsatter.com/shopping to purchase books and review other resources.

Schaefer, J. (2003) *Life Without Ed: How One Woman Declared Independence from Her Eating Disorder and How You Can Too*. New York, NY: McGraw-Hill.

Schaefer, J. (2009) *Goodbye Ed, Hello Me: Recover from Your Eating Disorder and Fall in Love with Life*. New York, NY: McGraw-Hill.

INDEX